No One
Ailing
Except a
Physician

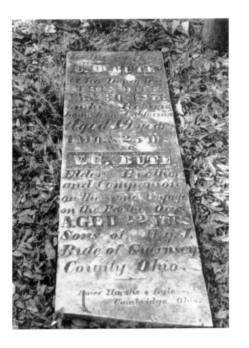

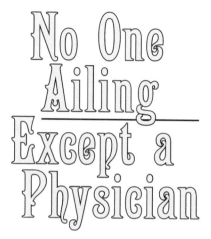

No One Ailing Except a Physician

Medicine in the Mining West, 1848–1919

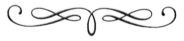

Duane A. Smith & Ronald C. Brown

University Press of Colorado
Boulder

Published by the University Press of Colorado
5589 Arapahoe Avenue, Suite 206C
Boulder, Colorado 80303

The University Press of Colorado is a cooperative publishing enterprise supported, in part, by Adams State University, Colorado State University, Fort Lewis College, Metropolitan State University of Denver, Regis University, University of Colorado, University of Northern Colorado, Utah State University, and Western State Colorado University.

The paper used in this publication meets the minimum requirements of the American National Standard for Information Sciences—Permanence of Paper for Printed Library Materials. ANSI Z39.48-1992

Library of Congress Cataloging-in-Publication Data

Brown, Ronald C., 1945–
    No one ailing except a physician : medicine in the mining West,
1848–1919 / Ronald C. Brown, Duane A. Smith.
       p. cm.
    Includes bibliographical references and index.
    ISBN 0-87081-611-X (alk. paper) — ISBN 978-1-60732-352-5 (pbk. : alk. paper)
    1. Medicine—West (U.S.)—History—19th century. I. Smith, Duane A. II. Title.
    R154.5.W47 B76 2001
    610'.978'09034—dc21
                                                                                    00-013225

Design by Daniel Pratt

 Co-winner of the 2000 Colorado Endowment for the Humanities Publication Prize

The CEH Publication Prize was created in 1998 and the first awards were made in 1999. The prize annually supports publication of outstanding nonfiction works that have strong humanities content and that make an area of humanities research more available to the Colorado public. The CEH Publication Prize funds are shared by the University Press of Colorado and the authors of the works being recognized.

    The Colorado Endowment for the Humanities is a statewide, nonprofit organization dedicated to improving the quality of humanities education for all Coloradans.

for
Judy and Gay
Lara and Brian

Contents

Preface

NINETEENTH- AND EARLY TWENTIETH-CENTURY MINING PEOPLE might have agreed with the "father of medicine," Hippocrates, when he wrote more than 2,000 years before, "Medicine is the most distinguished of all the arts, but through the ignorance of those who practice it, and of those who casually judge such practitioners, it is now of all the arts by far the least esteemed."

One has only to wander through a mining community cemetery to understand the high price people paid to work in the industry and to live in the camps and towns. Modern medicine was still several generations away. Thus, they were fated to doctor themselves or trust in the treatment and medicines of the local physician. The result was often only too predictable.

A book such as this is never solely the product of the author, or, in this case, the authors. We would like to thank the following colleagues and librarians for their assistance with research on this project. We owe special thanks to Gene Gressley of the University of Wyoming's American Heritage Center, Greg Thompson of the University of Utah Libraries, Margaret Vaverek of Texas State University, and Dr. Joseph Murphy who graciously read several chapters. The staffs of the Bancroft Library, the Huntington Library, Fort Lewis College Library, Arizona State University Library, Denver Public Library Western History Department, University of Colorado Library, Montana Historical Society, Nevada Historical Society, Deadwood Library, Homestake Mining Company, Wells Fargo Bank, and Texas State University Alkek Library were most helpful. There are others, over the decade of research and writing on this project, whose names, but not contributions, have been forgotten. Our thanks to one and all.

This volume is dedicated to our wives and children, who once again lost us as we immersed ourselves in mining and medicine of years gone by.

Prologue

"THE PAST IS NOT DEAD. IT LIVES ON."

I N 1848 AMERICANS WELCOMED THE INVIGORATING NEWS of gold discoveries in far-off California. Determined to share in the wealth, many
began the adventure of their lives the next spring. The fact that these
immigrants had attained an age that allowed them to venture west was the
result of a combination of good luck, good health, and a dose of medicine
we Americans five generations later cannot fully appreciate. "Modern
medicine" is astonishingly recent—90 percent of it dates from World War
II and after—although most Americans in the 1840s had a better knowledge
of medicine than they did of mining.

This is the story of the interrelationship of the two—western mining
and medicine—from that tumultuous year of 1848 through the tragic influenza epidemic of 1918–1919. Had these forty-niners known more about
mining, they might never have ventured west. They fervently believed they
would find their golden bonanzas. The opportunity was there for the taking, but success could not be guaranteed. Mining reporter Eliot Lord wrote
in the early 1880s, "Mining is, perhaps, the only business pursuit in which
men stake large fortunes on the acquisition of prizes against the balance
of probabilities. It is certainly the only business undertaking where skill,
energy, foresight, and industry, aided by ample capital, will not command
a measure of success."[1] The fact that the odds stayed long never deterred
these optimists, who rushed into one new mining district after another over
the next sixty years.

To do this with even a modicum of success, they had to remain healthy,
not an easy task considering the state of the medical profession in 1848. The
doctors—the front line—were not held in high repute and commanded little
respect. Ineffective and primitive treatments did little to inspire confidence
in patients, who often sought out their physicians only after all else had
failed. These prevailing conditions meant that illness too frequently resulted
in death or, more often, permanent disability or disfigurement.

In some areas, particularly the East, physicians glutted the market, leading to complaints that they were not able to make a living. Patients nevertheless howled about their high fees. In Vermont that fee was fifty cents and in Mississippi one dollar per visit unless one lived a mile beyond the office. At that point the price rose alarmingly, based on mileage and whether the call came during the night or day. The doctors had some justification for the rate differential during a time when country roads required extra time and trouble. Rural calls also took them out of their offices, making it difficult for other patients to locate them. So the complaints went on, and the profession suffered accordingly.

Calling it a profession stretched the definition of the term. All who had the inclination to dabble in medicine could hang out their shingles and declare themselves open for business. Those who had read a book about medicine, taken a course or a brief apprenticeship, or perhaps simply become intrigued by medicine could literally "practice" in this era of few licensing laws or medical regulations. Statistics from eastern states indicated that a high percentage (up to a quarter) of so-called physicians were totally unqualified to practice medicine; in the West the figure was even higher. Unfortunately, mainstream medical groups resisted efforts to improve standards of medical education for fear doing so might hurt them. As a result, "quacks" outnumbered credentialed physicians in some areas. Mark Twain wrote a few years later, "He has been a doctor a year now, and has had two patients—no, three, I think; yes, it *was* three. I attended their funerals."

The public perception of physicians was colored by self-interest and characterized by ambivalence. Medicine and medical treatments, then and now, struck at the heart of all people's concern for life and its preservation. The doctor-patient relationship generated both extreme fears and hopeful expectations, as well as self-deceptions and unfulfilled promises. Patients expected doctors to provide more than was humanly possible, and overly eager doctors sometimes promised more than they could deliver. The seeds of discontent had been sown; disenchantment with doctors stretched back for generations, and public confidence in the profession had been deteriorating for many years.

The Jacksonian era of material and social progress, with its free-wheeling individualism and expectations, produced a startling number of malpractice suits in the East. Doctors reacted with anger and fear, blaming much of the trend on lawyers looking for fat fees. That might have been a small factor, but it was a natural reaction in a generation that did not hold the status of the medical profession in high esteem and that blamed people and institutions for personal misfortune.[2]

Medical science shared the blame with doctors for the deplorable state of the profession. In the first half of the nineteenth century, medicine had hardly advanced beyond the realm of the ancient Greeks. In 1840, for example, at least thirty-eight schools of thought existed on the theory of disease. Medical diagnosis was unsystematic and superficial; a person's pulse, skin color, breathing, and appearance of urine were the primary factors in diagnosis. Heredity was seen as the principal precipitator of illness. Surgery was hazardous because of a lack of anesthetics and ignorance of the causes of infection. Most operations were performed at home because of the fear or unavailability of hospitals. Once considered almshouses or charity institutions, hospitals had the image of a place to die rather than be cured. In reality, most patients expected to be treated at home and to die in their own beds. Rural medicine lingered behind urban, then as now, leaving most Americans in a medical backwater. Dentistry stayed even more primitive. Tooth extraction, utilized by blacksmiths, doctors, and home practitioners, constituted the panacea for most dental ailments.

Doctors needed resourcefulness and imagination to find medications that would ease a patient's ills. They prescribed opium (for pain and diarrhea), quinine (malaria), mercury (syphilis), and morphine (dysentery) with casual indifference to side effects. Purgatives and emetics were widely used, with calomel (mercurous chloride) the most popular, a stock-in-trade for laity and physician alike. Calomel, the aspirin of the nineteenth century, was hailed in medical journals as the "Sampson of the materia medica." Physicians prescribed that "therapeutic mule," arsenic, for a variety of external and internal problems from rheumatism to syphilis. Bloodletting even lingered as a curative in some areas. Questions were raised about the curative claims of these practices by the second half of the nineteenth century, but that did not stop their use. Some physicians used whiskey as an antiseptic, others as a crude anesthetic. A few lavished it on their insides to steady their nerves.

Medicine's sorry situation often forced Americans to turn to home remedies rather than to physicians, a strategy that potentially only made matters worse. Considering the state of medicine, the choice was understandable. Drinking sulphur was thought to be good for almost anything, as were quinine, calomel, black pepper, mustard plasters, and strong teas. Morphine and laudanum (tincture of opium) brought relief for pain, and the latter could also cure inflammation. Belladonna acted as a stimulant. Powdered drugs such as these could be purchased in a drug store or from a doctor for stocking one's personal medicine chest. Wood ashes or cobwebs stopped bleeding, and a bag of asafetida worn around the neck cured a cold.[3]

Many Americans, if they could afford private treatment, chose it in preference to a hospital stay. That decision was easy to understand. Cleanliness did not constitute a virtue in the hospital setting; patients, especially children, routinely fell victim to other diseases while hospitalized, and trained nurses (men) were seldom available. The quality of hospital staffs proved uneven, even according to the standards of the day, and they often worked under abominable conditions. Public hospitals were seen as refuges for the poor and even private hospitals as a last medical resort for others. Improvement, fortunately, loomed around the corner because of Florence Nightingale's work in the Crimean War and developments resulting from the U.S. Civil War. But like everything else, reform and modernization would come slowly.

In the 1840s anesthesia made significant strides when nitrous oxide, ether, and chloroform came into use. Before these advances the surgeon's most desirable skill had been his speed in performing surgical procedures. The number of operations increased when patients suffered less traumatic shock and pain, although results did not necessarily improve.

The reader should not make too much of or condemn too vehemently the misconceptions, ineffective procedures, and confusion of our nineteenth-century medical forebears. Within the era in which they lived, they were doing the best they knew how with the knowledge, equipment, techniques, and medicines available.

The American public harbored a certain fatalism about the practice of medicine. This was, after all, the generation that championed the individual. None was more individualistic than the western miner and the mining camp denizen. As a Virginia City physician phrased it, "Whoever wishes to go to the dogs, goes to the dogs. There is no restraint, or, as they express it, 'There is nobody holding you.'"

Americans complicated the health picture by failing to take good care of themselves, especially if such care hindered their scramble for cherished wealth. Forty-niner physician James L. Tyson expressed the prevailing attitude: "But who is careful or who is prudent in the pursuit of gold in California?" After the investigative work of Scotsman James Lind in the mid-eighteenth century, the concept of eating oranges, lemons, and limes to prevent and cure scurvy had become well understood. The ingestion of cream of tartar and vinegar, according to popular belief, also combatted the dietary deficiency that caused scurvy. Yet the forty-niners, in their rush to riches, ignored common wisdom (eating fresh fruit and vegetables) and medical counsel. They paid a severe penalty. Americans were some of the best-fed people in the world in 1849; nevertheless, scurvy stalked them relentlessly. They had no one to blame but themselves.[4]

Other examples of the materialistic, cavalier attitude toward health and quality of life included a lack of attention to sanitation and failure to prevent and control epidemics. Mining community folks were not alone in disregarding the common sense and medical wisdom of the day; Americans from the East Coast to the West shared their guilt. The popular *Gunn's*

Domestic Medicine expressed what the comic strip character Pogo would say years later: "Among the moral causes that have abridged the life of man, there is one which merits the attention of the philosopher—it is civilization!" In Pogo's words, "The enemy is us."

Impatience also handicapped mulish Americans in their pursuit of good health. A doctor's wife, S. Anna Gordon, accurately summarized the problem in the late 1870s when she recounted a trip to Colorado:

> Educated as our American people are to the idea that everything must be done in a hurry, travelling has not been made an exception to this general rule. We, as a nation, work in a hurry; we sleep in a hurry. . . . We live in a hurry, wear out the machinery of life in a hurry, and die prematurely.

Western mining people exemplified this characteristic to the ultimate degree. They spent their whole lives rushing to catch yesterday before it became tomorrow, a frantic chase for the pot of gold at the end of the rainbow.

There is much to be learned about these people and what motivated them in a study of medicine and western mining. It is a window to yesteryear and a mirror for today. As scholar and educator George Norlin wrote, "The past is not dead. It lives on in our speech, our habits, our thoughts, our institutions."[5]

Notes

1. John Steele Gordon, "How America's Health Care Fell Ill," *American Heritage* (May-June 1992), 49, 52; Eliot Lord, *Comstock Mining and Miners* (Washington, D.C.: Government Printing Office, 1883), 360.

2. Sources for this section are Martin Kaufman, *American Medical Education* (Westport, Conn.: Greenwood, 1976), 93, 101; Billy M. Jones, *Health-Seekers in the Southwest, 1817–1900* (Norman: University of Oklahoma Press, 1967), 23, 26; John S. Haller Jr., *American Medicine in Transition 1840–1910* (Urbana: University of Illinois Press, 1981), chapters 3 and 4; Paul Starr, *The Social Transformation of American Medicine* (New York: Basic, 1982), 64, 66–68, 82–83, 145–147, 154–155; James G. Burrow, *AMA: Voice of American Medicine* (Baltimore: Johns Hopkins University Press, 1963), 1–3, 8–9; George Groh, "Doctors of the Frontier," *American Heritage* (April 1963), 11; Richard Dunlap, *Doctors of the American Frontier* (New York: Doubleday, 1965), 4; Mark Twain, *The Gilded Age* (New York: Harper and Brothers, 1915), 102; Robert F. Karolevitz, *Doctors of the Old West* (Seattle: Superior, 1967), 65; David Malmsheimer, "Doctors Only," in *The Evolving Image of the American Physician* (New York: Greenwood, 1988), 11–12, 16, 18; Kenneth A. De Ville, *Medical Malpractice in Nineteenth-Century America* (New York: New York University Press, 1990), 25–27, 64–65, 89–90, 115, 122, 137.

3. Gordon, "How America's Health Care Fell Ill," 51; William G. Rothstein, *American Medical Schools and the Practice of Medicine* (New York: Oxford Uni-

versity Press, 1987), 39–41, 73–75; James H. Cassedy, *Medicine in America: A Short History* (Baltimore: Johns Hopkins University Press, 1991), 44–51, 53–58; Geoffrey Marks and William K. Beatty, *The Story of Medicine in America* (New York: Charles Scribner's Sons, 1973), 198–202; Jake W. Spidle, *Doctors of Medicine in New Mexico* (Albuquerque: University of New Mexico Press, 1986), 79–80; Groh, "Doctors of the Frontier," 10; Clarence Meyer, *American Folk Medicine* (New York: Thomas Y. Crowell, 1973), 14–15; Karolevitz, *Doctors of the Old West*, 139, 169–170; Haller, *American Medicine*, 87–89, 90–91, 98.

4. Kenneth M. Ludmerer, *Learning to Heal* (Baltimore: Johns Hopkins University Press, 1985), 9–12; Rothstein, *American Medical Schools*, 77–78, 85–86; Gordon, "How America's Health Care Fell Ill," 51; Charles Shinn, *The Story of the Mine* (New York: D. Appleton, 1898), 240; James L. Tyson, *Diary of a Physician in California* (Oakland: Biobooks, 1955 reprint), 77; Kenneth J. Carpenter, *The History of Scurvy and Vitamin C* (Cambridge: Cambridge University Press, 1986), 51–52, 95–96, 98, 101; Joseph R. Conlin, *Bacon, Beans, and Galantines* (Reno: University of Nevada Press, 1986), 6, 72, 74.

5. John C. Gunn, *Gunn's Domestic Medicine* (Xenia, Ohio: J. H. Purdy, 1837), 2; S. Anna Gordon, *Camping in Colorado* (New York: Authors' Publishing, 1879), 21; Ralph E. Ellsworth, ed., *A Voice From Colorado's Past for the Present: Selected Writings of George Norlin* (Boulder: Colorado Associated Press, 1985), 55.

No One
Ailing
Except a
Physician

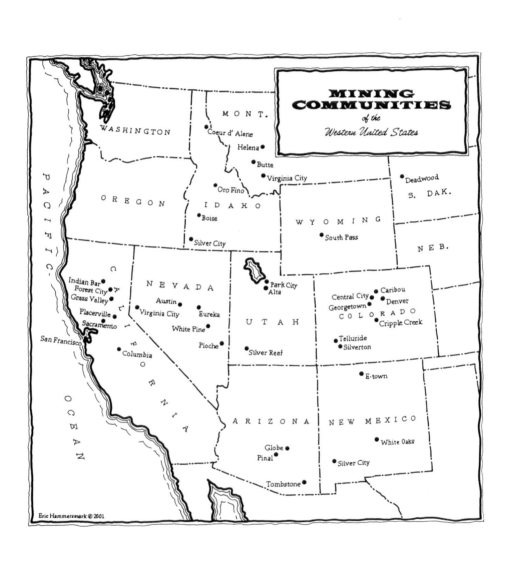

MINING
COMMUNITIES
of the
Western United States

1

"Life and Death Jostle Each Other"

CALIFORNIA'S GOLD RUSH ERA

THE YEAR, 1848; THE MONTH, JANUARY; the site, a sawmill under construction for Swiss émigré John Sutter on the south fork of the American River. Back in August 1847, Sutter had contracted with drifter and jack-of-all trades James Marshall to carry out the project. Now it came to an unexpected climax.

On the morning of the twenty-fourth, Marshall ventured out to inspect the newly exposed bed of the tailrace. The astonished carpenter saw what he believed to be gold scattered along the bed. He showed the samples to his workers, conducted a few crude tests, and several days later rode down to Sutter's Fort, where Sacramento would soon be located. After conducting his own tests, Sutter was convinced gold had been discovered. Fearing that his dream of a California empire would be threatened, he attempted to keep the news under wraps—to no avail.

The news that gold had been discovered in California would soon make its way around the world; the nineteenth century's greatest gold rush was poised on the starting blocks. Few participants grasped its global significance. Most saw it as their best chance to make a fortune or at the least to achieve a more comfortable way of life than they had ever experienced. The opportunity to "get rich without working" has been irresistible to fortune seekers in all centuries.

The first wave of interest swelled slowly. San Francisco's *California Star* noted inconspicuously on March 18, 1848, amid comments about quicksilver, copper, and silver mines, that gold had been discovered about "40 miles above Sutter's Fort." Nine weeks later the newspaper featured the latest highly flattering accounts from the gold country—so flattering that San Francisco felt the first impact of the excitement. "Stores are closed and places of business vacated; a large number of houses tenantless, various kinds of mechanical labor suspended or given up entirely, and nowhere the pleasant hum of industry salutes the ear of late." On June 14 the *Star* itself stopped publishing; more important matters lured the staff and its readers to the Sierras.[1]

Already a "motley assemblage, composed of lawyers, merchants, grocers, carpenters, and cooks, all possessed with the desire of becoming suddenly rich," had rushed to the mines. From San Francisco to Los Angeles, the word spread. Soon would-be miners came in from Washington and Oregon, then from Mexico and South America. As early as August, reports of riches reached the eastern states, but several months passed before "the golden yellow fever" caught hold there. By winter the news had reached England and Europe, and the stage was set for the great 1849 gold rush.

They planned and dreamed, these soon-to-be forty-niners. They saw the chance of a lifetime unfolding before them. In the words of the popular song "Ho! For California!":

> As we explore that distant shore—
> We'll fill our pockets with the shining ore;
> And how 'twill sound, as the word goes round,
> Of our picking up gold by the dozen pound.

Many forty-eighters were already finding the bonanzas about which they had dreamed. Edward Gould Buffum was one of those who reached the diggings in the fall of 1848. His party on Weaver's Creek averaged about an ounce ($20) a day per individual, excellent wages indeed compared with the $1 per eleven-hour day an ordinary laborer might earn back in the states. As commonly occurred in the turmoil of the times, Buffum got wind of better diggings to the north, packed up, and left, leaving his older claim "for some other digger to work out." The new diggings paid off handsomely—he found a pocket of gold containing over twenty-nine ounces. For a few hours work, Buffum made more money than many Americans did in a year.

Rev. Walter Colton toured the mines that same fall and reported that a man he knew brought out $5,356 worth of gold after sixty-four days. And so the stories went. The truth proved wonderful enough at the time, but the farther from California the tales traveled, the more they gained in the retelling. Young Lt. William T. Sherman was more cautious when writing from Sutter's Fort in October: "It is impossible to get at anything like the truth, but that the amount of gold in these mountains exceeds any previous calculation I have no doubt." Not all profits were clear, however; the miners found the cost of living in the isolated canyons and rivers higher than anywhere they had previously lived or mined. Stories of the downside of the California rush traveled much less quickly![2]

In 1849, the wonderful year of the California gold rush, Americans rushed to "see the elephant." Gold fever hit the young, middle-aged, and old alike. Other states claimed their share of the excitement with reports of gold in New Jersey, Texas, Michigan, Maryland, and elsewhere. Some sought to dampen enthusiasm and quell the rush. The *Placer Times* forecast that of the many who went in search of gold, "few will return" and those "few not much richer than before."

At least one prospective bride was left standing at the altar, and a young man rejected his mother's offer of $20,000 if he would stay home. That amount looked like small potatoes compared with the value of the nuggets he had been reading about. Americans traveled by steamer, sailing ship, and overland wagons beginning in early 1849. Foreigners—Englishmen, Mexicans, Irishmen, Frenchmen, Australians, Chinese, South Americans—rushed to the Sierra Nevadas to try their luck and skill in a huge golden lottery. Whether by sea or land, the trip proved arduous, yet a hundred thousand people, give or take a few, reached California. Neither the United States nor the world had ever seen anything like this, and they never would again. The significance of this rush redounded to the following decades, well past the turn of the twentieth century.

The Argonauts ventured west, intending to make their fortunes and return home within a season or two at most. What they found was that placer gold (free gold found in streams or in former stream channels) did exist, sometimes in unbelievable amounts, but that the 1848ers had already preempted the best of it:

> When I got there, the mining ground
> Was staked and claimed for miles around,
> And not a bed was to be found,
> When I went off to prospect.

Thus sang the forlorn prospector in the contemporary folk song "When I Went off to Prospect." Not riches but ill health was a more common product of intensive labor. There were songs about that, too:

> I got into the water, where the "fever-n-ager" took me,
> And after I was froze to death, it turned about and shook me;
> But still I kept to work, a hopin' 'twould be better,
> But the water wouldn't fall a bit, but kept a getting wetter.[3]

The one-time farmers, merchants, seamen, teachers, doctors, ministers, soldiers, or whatever found out the reality of what a later miner confessed: "I never worked so hard in my life to get rich without working."

The toil exacted a terrible toll on the miners and prospectors. The cost in human lives and ruined health just to reach California had been appalling. Far more migrants died of disease while crossing the continent than were killed by Indians. They were the first but not the last to discover the exorbitant cost of following the sordid cry "gold, gold, GOLD!"

The route an individual took to travel west determined which diseases he or she might encounter or succumb to. None proved disease free. The quickest trip for Americans (with luck, five weeks), and the most expensive, lay through the Isthmus of Panama. This fever-ridden journey killed thousands and left many more forty-niners debilitated when they arrived in California. Malaria could kill them along the Chagres River or attack them later with the same result. The ship route around Cape Horn and up the west coast of South America was long and wearisome, taking four to eight months. Spoiled food, cramped quarters, seasickness, impure water, boredom, unsanitary conditions, and inactivity brought the would-be miners into San Francisco harbor in poor physical condition.[4]

The overland trail from the Missouri River to the West Coast was in some ways the most rugged, but it kept the Argonauts outdoors, a distinct advantage. Along the well-known Oregon Trail and the California cutoff lurked a number of unanticipated dangers. The lucky parties made the trip in five months, others needed seven or eight.

No matter how fast the immigrants traveled, they could not outrun cholera, the great killer of 1849–1850. The forty-niners called cholera "the ruthless destroyer," and one described the road from Independence, Missouri, to Fort Laramie as a "graveyard." The disease had made its way from Europe to New Orleans in 1848 and quickly spread up the Mississippi Valley. Now it found its way onto the plains. Interestingly, it inexplicably abated beyond Fort Laramie, perhaps because of the higher altitude, fresh water, and less congestion among the emigrant trains. Other aliments lay in wait, however, as cholera receded.

The cause of this dreaded disease remained a mystery in 1849. Indeed, a popular medical book, *Gunn's Domestic Medicine* (1837), after describing the suspected cause and the preferred treatment, concluded, "Suffer me to remind you of one important preventive in this epidemic: at all times and under all circumstances, to place a reliance upon Almighty God." Pioneers had a saying about cholera that revealed a great deal about attitudes toward the medical profession as well.

> Cholera kills and doctors slay,
> and every foe will have its way.

Dr. Israel Lord treated his patients along the trail with a "single dose of laudanum, with pepper, camphor, musk, ammonia, peppermint or other stimulants" and claimed a cure in a few minutes. On another wagon train Dr. Charles Parke prescribed "Hyd. Choloite, capsicum and camphor," along with opium. His patient recovered. Generally, the disease struck suddenly, and death came within hours, usually after "great agony."

Fevers of various kinds, many carried by the pioneers from their midwestern homes, wreaked havoc all along the trail. The forty-niners listed lung, camp, typhus, bilious, typhoid, and the ever-popular ague as fever ailments. Mountain fever, a term the gold rushers used loosely to describe almost any fever that struck them in or near the mountains, would also be a factor in the later Pike's Peak rush (it was probably Rocky Mountain Spotted or Colorado Tick Fever). Fort Kearny's post physician wrote in August 1858 that he "never saw as much malaria and fever and ague as there was in the trains from the East." Known by various terms—fever, ague, chills, intermittent or remittent fever—the ailments all generally referred to malaria.

Overlander Mary Bailey referred to her husband's hard chill—and to herself as sick and tired. The constant travel exhausted animals and humans; the physical exertion required of both to reach California was staggering. Catching a fever in this situation, far from home and civilized comforts, leant a new meaning to the word *sickness*.[5]

Dr. John Hudson Wyman, who crossed the Oregon Trail in 1852, reported that both diarrhea and dysentery had invaded his train. Scurvy ranked as the third major killer after cholera and mountain fever, becoming prevalent, especially in the later stages of a trail journey, after months on a diet of salt pork and flapjacks. Some mistook its early stages for rheumatism, but eventually there was no mistaking it. One Californian observed train after train arriving in late 1849 and described what he saw as follows: "A more pitiable sight I had never before beheld. There were cripples from scurvy—children who could not move a limb."

The forty-niners suffered from scurvy more than any other group that had ever rushed to a new bonanza and seemingly had no one to blame but themselves. Neither those who hurried to the earlier Georgia and North Carolina discoveries nor the 1848ers found scurvy a significant problem in their camps despite a similar frenzy in seeking gold and not worrying about food. To be sure, they had not traveled as far, and the southern miners had a good food base, but once in camp the situation nearly equaled 1849 conditions. Only the Klondike rushers of 1898 experienced similar problems.

On the trail, more ordinary illnesses such as mumps, rheumatism, measles, bilious complaints, "summer complaints," and even the common cold created unusual complications. Smallpox was a dreaded scourge. Pregnancy's inherent stresses and dangers became more perilous. A toothache could progress to something more than a mere annoyance. The always perceptive Louise Clapp (family spelling) wrote from Indian Bar, California, in October 1852 that hardly any families had not buried a beloved member on the plains. The poor women arrive, she concluded, looking as haggard as "many Endorean witches."

The physicians and pseudo-physicians who traveled west among the rushers understood little of the causes or cures of most of these diseases. Dr. E. A. Tompkins came up with some possible explanations in 1850. He first blamed the high saline and alkaline content of the water and the ingestion of fish before hitting closer to the mark when he pointed to poor preparation of camp food, chilly night watches, sleeping on cold wet ground, and finally, the "constant hard and exhausting toil." If doctors were ignorant of causes and cures, the rest of the Argonauts could hardly be expected to cope with the multitude of illnesses they had rarely or never before encountered.[6]

When they arrived in California, the forty-niners threw themselves into learning the work of mining. The physical toil and stress involved in reaching the goldfields had undermined many of their constitutions at the time when a new lifestyle and hard labor demanded strength and endurance. Sacramento's *Placer Times* (December 8, 1849) summarized the situation concisely when it referred to mining on the Yuba River. The editor said one rarely heard of an individual's not doing well "if he has been able to preserve his health."

Miner Alonzo Delano, who wrote several books and many newspaper articles about his experiences, observed in March 1850 that most immigrants, even if they arrived in good health, would "be sick after arrival." He concluded, "Exposure and bad diet contribute much to producing sickness." Contemporary William Swain concurred: "Exposure causes sickness to a great extent, for in most of the mines tents are all the habitation miners have." Delano pointed out another factor involved in ill health when he wrote that many immigrants "rushed to the mine and went to work . . . without blankets to shield them from the cold night air."

California's climate had garnered a reputation for being salubrious, but the miners found the mountains, although invigorating much of the time, decidedly miserable during the rainy winter season. Damp, cold, sunless days for weeks on end could make mining in and along the streams physical torture. Standing and stooping in the cold, muddy water even on warm days involved tough manual labor. Yet the miners believed they must continue to work even in the worst conditions. Daniel Woods explained why:

> This morning [January 15, 1850], notwithstanding the rain, we were again at our work. We must work. In sunshine and rain, in warm and cold, in sickness and health, successful or not successful, early and late, it is work, *work*, WORK! *Work or Perish!* All around us, above and below, on mountainside and stream, the rain falling fast upon them, are the miners at work—not for *gold*, but for *bread*.

Friedrich Gerstaecker complained that clothes had no time to "dry thoroughly on our bodies," and such a life was sufficient to "shake the strongest constitution besides being [as] unpleasant as any one could desire."[7]

In the heat of summer, some of these inconveniences abated, but the glare of the sun, the sharp contrast between cold water work and warm land life, and the generally unsanitary conditions of the camps and placer mines led to different health problems. Fleas and lice commonly accompanied the miners. For many, neatness and cleanliness did not equate to godliness in the realm of personal hygiene, laundering, and housekeeping.

Louise Clapp described littered Indian Bar: "The whole Bar is thickly peppered with empty bottles, oyster cans, sardine boxes and brandied fruit jars." The forty-niners and their descendants scattered trash with utter disregard for aesthetics or environmental consequences. This was only a temporary home that would be left behind without a second look. They intended to return east once they made their "pile" or stampede off to a more promising discovery. Clapp decided that miners were the "most discontented of mortals" who would wander off in search of better diggings even when their current claim was paying steady dividends.

Along with the work and the climate, the miners' diet undermined their health. Compounding the problem were shortages of food and high transportation costs, exacerbated by seasonal rain and snow, which ultimately translated into increased food prices. Those conditions dampened the incentive to seek out variety or balance in food intake. After long hours of work, it was too much of a chore and took too much time to plan, purchase, and cook what today would be termed a balanced meal. The daily menu comprised beans, bread, and beef. Scotsman J. D. Borthwick described his bill of fare as "beefsteaks, damper [flour/water dough] and tea"—morning, noon, and night. Many years later, forty-niner R. C. Shaw remembered that he ate "stewed beans and flapjacks 21 times per week though the latter was occasionally replaced by flour dumplings and molasses." Dr. Jacob D.B. Stillman lamented that in Sacramento in 1850 he had "almost forgotten what I used to eat at home."[8]

Disappointed dreams, homesickness, and moods wildly fluctuating between optimism and depression conspired to produce an unhealthy mental environment among the gold seekers. Some collapsed under the stress or suffered from "temporary insanity." Those who could not regain control usually found themselves in a state asylum. The sick miner needed a friend; lacking one, he sometimes died, as Stillman wrote, on the ground, "unknown, unconscious, uncared for."

Merchant/miner John Ingalls blamed the adverse conditions for the fact that "there are thousands of persons here who hardly ever saw a sick day in the States and are completely broken-down, and many of them, if they live, will never fully recover their health." Physician James Tyson concurred, observing that few of those who worked the mines left with their accustomed health: "I never saw so many broken-down constitutions as during my brief stay in California."

Scurvy became one of the worst scourges of 1849–1850, bringing down many already weakened forty-niners. Edward Gould Buffum testified that at least half the miners he knew were stricken. He came down with it himself and nearly died, leaving behind a graphic account of his suffering:

> [I experienced] swelling and bleeding of the gums, followed by a swelling of both legs below the knee, which rendered me unable to walk. For three weeks I was obliged to feed upon the very articles that had caused the disease and growing daily weaker, enduring the most intense suffering from pain in my limbs which were now becoming more swollen and turning black.

He was saved by some beans a friend found growing wild and a decoction of the bark of the spruce tree. Both the symptoms and the treatment were typical of that era. Others consumed a tea made of sassafras and spruce leaves, acidulous drinks, stewed fruits, and pickles. The lack of fresh vegetables and fruits lay at the root of this diet-deficiency disease, but it was abetted, at least among the seafaring forty-niners, by the sudden physical exertion now required.

Burying live scurvy victims in the earth up to their necks was not a typical remedy! Some camps interred all but a few of their residents in that manner in an attempt to halt an epidemic. The unburied few stood guard to "keep off grizzlys and coyotes." The effectiveness of this procedure was not recorded, but after 1850 nothing more was heard of scurvy epidemics.

The high prices the miners were eventually willing to pay for a varied diet caused freighters and merchants to offer an increased supply of vegetables, fruits, oranges, and limes. In Grass Valley, California, in the winter of 1853–1854, for instance, peaches, limes, apples, potatoes, cherries, and dates enticed customers. At first glance it seems inconceivable that scurvy could have been rampant in California, the land of milk and honey. But this soon-to-be state had not yet begun to produce large amounts of vegetables, fruits, and grain. Transportation remained costly, slow, and hampered by weather, and many miners had no knowledge of what wild plants could be used to alleviate their symptoms.

Scurvy, which may or may not have been the worst affliction, had many equally debilitating companions. Dr. James Tyson ranked rheumatism and dysentery along with scurvy. In the second half of 1850, the State Marine Hospital in San Francisco admitted 262 patients with diarrhea, 204 with dysentery, 160 with rheumatism, and 93 with "intermittent fever." The appearance of fevers was not unexpected, caused as they were by conditions in the mines and complicated by the Argonauts' state when they arrived. Stillman observed that in Sacramento in November 1849, diarrhea was so general that "it has been popularly regarded as the disease of California . . . with the number of deaths greater than from any other disease." Also, as the *Alta California* (August 30, 1849) pointed out, many feared an attack of diarrhea was the "precursor of the terrible scourge cholera."

Surprisingly, cholera did not make its debut until 1850, by which time many believed Californians led a charmed existence. That confidence was contradicted when the scourge returned in 1852 and 1854. Smallpox created no cause for concern as an epidemic. Those miners who encountered poison oak remembered it as something far more discomforting than dooming. Local remedies soothed the suffering, and it is hoped that one suggestion was rejected out of hand—chewing the poison oak leaves without swallowing them!

Alcoholism claimed victims from the beginning of the rush. Failure, boredom, the overwhelmingly masculine society, a lack of homes, stress, and the climate aided and abetted consumption of "demon rum." Californians acquired an unsavory reputation for excessive drinking, which caused its own health problems and complicated those already in existence. Hard drinking endured as one of the legends of the forty-niners and was one of the most prevalent medical problems in the mining West.[9]

Where could the miners turn for help in alleviating illness and discomfort? The reputation of doctors sank to new lows in the mining camps. To quote a common saying, "Cholera may come now and then, but doctors are always with us." The high fees doctors charged in the mining regions led most men to rely on their own or their companions' devices. Eventually, regardless of the cost, many visited a doctor. Toothaches bedeviled Henry Page for four months in 1850. He tried first to allay the pain with pipe tobacco, then sought out a doctor, who failed to pull the offending tooth. He finally went to Sacramento, where a physician extracted it with little trouble. Another ache appeared and another tooth was pulled, prompting him to write his wife that "if it keeps on this rate you will have a toothless, bald old man for a husband."

William Swain, who mined on the south fork of the Feather River, came down with chills, fever, and dysentery. From the medicines he had with him he "took opium and a large dose of quinine, which checked the disease." Several days later, however, he suffered a relapse:

> I was not well next morning: took physic. That afternoon had some
> fever, the same the two following days but no chills. There was not
> apparently anything the matter with me, but my strength was all gone. I

knew not what to do and called a doctor, who examined me and told us
that my disease was subdued and all that was needed was strengthening.

The doctor dosed Swain with some powders, followed by drops of tincture
of iron and dogwood bitters for two weeks. He eventually recovered. Swain
provided a case study of a successful combination of home remedies and a
doctor's advice.

Many Argonauts had brought medicines with them; the customary
precaution was to take along a medicine chest containing a trusted assortment of home remedies. Catherine Haun's "portable apothecary shop"
included quinine for malaria, citric acid for scurvy, hartshorn for snakebite,
and "bluemass" (a compound made of mercury, honey, and some wax or
other malleable substance), opium, and whiskey for almost everything else.
Another chest included some of these same items, as well as a box of physicking pills (laxative), castor oil, rum, and a vial of "peppermint essence."
Brandy, chloroform, laudanum, sulphur pills, morphine, and poultices made
with red pepper and mustard also had disciples. Patent medicines captured
their devotees; more than a few forty-niners brought bottles of potions
recommended by "specialists" or the "medical profession."

Opium and its derivatives topped the list of palliatives. One medical
book termed opium "the monarch of medical powers, the soothing angel
of moral and physical pain." Englishman Frank Marryat became anxious
when he saw too many gold seekers dosing themselves with another popular
nostrum, mercury. He believed quinine and castor oil were the only valu-
able medicines, but the ultimate answer to most ills was rest. That solution
created a dilemma for some men because, as he observed, "the fear of the
jeers of his healthier companions will often cause a man to continue to
work when prudence would dictate an opposite course."[10]

If all else failed, a visit to the doctor was the last resort. From the
very start of the rush, Sacramento's *Placer Times* carried physicians' advertisements (seven by early August 1849). Henry Bates, MD, for example,
advertised a hospital at Coloma (Sutter's Mill) where all the excitement
first erupted. Besides being near the mining districts, it offered, according
to the doctor, a "delightful view of the country," excellent spring water, and
his personal attention to all patients.

Prohibitive doctors' fees discouraged many miners. One disgusted
forty-niner summed up the attitude: "Dierea, piles, gravel, chills, fever and
scurvy begin to make their appearance and I ain't well myself. . . . There
has been three doctors or things they call doctors working at me for some
time. . . . Have now paid out all my gold to the doctors and they leave me
worse in health." Another complained that "the doctors charge pretty well.
They charge for pills as if they were diamonds, and bleed a man of an ounce

of gold and an ounce of blood at the same time." Operations that ranged as high as $1,000 did not enhance the profession's reputation.

The doctors had their side of the situation. Dr. John Wyman wrote his brother from Forest City in April 1855: "I can do a business amounting to at least $8,000 in a year, but probably could not collect more than one half, if that. There are so many destitute Creatures that you Can't make it Come out right." At least one Angels Camp physician was driven to desperation: "All persons knowing themselves indebted to the undersigned will please call & settle at least a portion of their indebtedness, as I am much in need of money." Some physicians found themselves unable to make ends meet and turned to such things as freighting, running board-inghouses, bartending, and running businesses (drug stores particularly) to supplement their incomes. Some mined and practiced while others practiced and mined, the ratio determined by how tenaciously gold fever had seized their souls.

About 1,300 to 1,500 doctors, or those self-proclaimed as such, were swept from east to west by the gold rush. A few, the Chinese for instance, migrated from west to east. They were a motley group—no question of credentials or medical association standards cluttered their consciences. Medical anarchy resulted.

> Each druggist clerk, who comes from the States,
> "Sets up" in the bleeding profession,
> If he kills a man, that he's called too late,
> Is excuse for the quackish transgression.

Thus concluded a bitter verse from the contemporary song "California Humbugs." Dr. Fayette Clapp found out the reality of the situation when he arrived at Rich Bar. He found two or three doctors there on his arrival, but in less than three weeks that number had increased to "*twenty-nine* who had chosen this place for the express purpose of practicing their profession."

At their best, doctors were well trained in a respectable school, such as Jacob Stillman of New York's College of Physicians and Surgeons. At their worst, they were quacks who hung out their shingles in hopes of making a fast buck. Howard Gardiner's 1854 problems exemplified the horrors of malpractice. Suffering from "excruciating" pain, he sent for a doctor who "pronounced the case one of inflammation of the prostate gland." The prescribed medicine had no effect, and poor Gardiner was reduced to swallowing large amounts of opium to kill the pain. "Disgusted with the doctors, I procured a copy of *Gunn's Domestic Medicine* and diagnosed my own case, a fistula in ano [anal abscess]." A subsequent examination by another physician proved his diagnosis correct, but now he needed an operation followed by a month's recuperation to recover.

A camp with a doctor (many never had even one) was an important attraction, even though the medical facility rarely resembled the imposing structures reminiscent of life in the states. After her husband launched his practice, Louise Clapp described his office, one some locals perceived as a special place, in this way:

> When I entered this imposing place, the shock to my optic nerves was so great that I sank, helplessly, upon one of the benches which ran, divan-like, the whole length (ten feet!) of the building, and laughed till I cried. There was, of course, no floor; a rude nondescript in one corner, on which was ranged the medical library, consisting of half a dozen volumes, did duty as a table. The shelves, which looked like sticks snatched hastily from the wood-pile and nailed up without the least alteration, contained quite a respectable array of medicines.

When Dr. Clapp endeavored to conduct a postmortem on two men, he could find no building that admitted enough light, so he held it out-of-doors. This proved a popular attraction for the "Kanakas, Indians, French, Spanish, English, Irish, and Yankees, who had gathered eagerly about the spot."[11]

The physicians practiced an eclectic variety of medicine, from age-old Chinese herbal remedies to the latest procedures from European and U.S. medical schools. Bleeding, which was losing favor in the East, was still popular among miners to relieve headaches, fevers, insanity, and infections. The medical arsenal of frontier doctors might have been limited, but they had that miracle drug, quinine, at the ready. Although the new wonders of anesthesia, ether, and chloroform were not available, the old standbys of whiskey and opium served the same purpose.

At their finest, physicians surmounted the limitations imposed on them with a combination of practical observation, devotion, and intelligence. James Tyson represented one of the best of the breed. In a book written in 1850, he proffered some suggestions to potential miners and older professionals about their health and occupation. He felt confident that these ideas would provide personal comfort, protection from diseases, and improved health generally:

> Do not work in the heat of the day, work two hours earlier in morning and in late afternoon.
>
> Relax occasionally from the stooping posture of mining.
>
> Cleanliness should never be neglected and frequent bathing provides an essential benefit.
>
> The quality of and preparation of food affects not only health but the miner's very life. Exclusive use of dried and salted meats is highly prejudicial. [He concluded with suggestions about what should be eaten.]

Whether many people followed Tyson's well-thought-out advice is not known, but at least this member of the medical profession had come to grips with some of the basic issues of health and illness in the mines. Unfortunately, his ideas would have stolen time from the basic hunt for wealth, an unacceptable compromise to ore seekers unwilling to act until sickness forced them to do so.

When it became obvious that permanent settlement was evolving from the transitory, individualized California placer mining era, medical leaders, as did others, attempted to institute the professional standards that existed in their eastern U.S. and ethnic homes. They endeavored to weed out doctors like Placerville's Dr. Hullings, who was said to be competent enough when sober, a rare occasion. He was eventually killed in a duel. The charlatans and quacks had to go, but the process was easier to preach than to practice.

In the 1850s medical leaders attempted to form local societies of doctors; some prospered briefly, only to fail within ten years. Permanent organization was not achieved until the late 1860s. Only Sacramento and San Francisco provided adequate hospitals during the first decade after the gold rush. Religious, private, and public hospitals accepted patients but did not guarantee cleanliness and adequate facilities. Communities cooperated in attempts to acquire better facilities and treatment. Sacramento and Placerville, for instance, created a Board of Health, or "hospital and sick" committees, and instituted health ordinances. The intentions, here and elsewhere, probably were better than any real ability to solve the problems.

Although this was a male-dominated rush and a masculine world, more women came every year. Louise Clapp tells poignantly of the sickness and death of Nancy Ann Bailey in isolated Rich Bar. The other three women in the camp went to the family's aid, but the tragedy could not be easily alleviated. The death of a mother and wife had a much greater impact on daily life in a camp than that of a single miner. A woman had no chance of finding a doctor of her own gender in those early days. Advertisements for women doctors rarely appeared in the press, although a few were published in 1854. The first regularly college-graduated woman doctor to come to California, Elizer Stone, arrived in 1857. During the entire gold rush period and for years afterward, women were forced to rely on male doctors, midwives, neighbors, or themselves.[12]

America's greatest placer gold rush was over. Indeed, by the early 1850s the golden days of '48 and '49 were being remembered in a hazy, romantic afterglow. An editorial in the *Marysville Herald*, August 20, 1850, did not gild the truth:

The people have been to each other strangers in a strange land. Absorbed in the eager pursuit of wealth, they have not taken time for the cultivation of those affinities which bind man to man by a higher and holier tie than mere interest. Their hearts have been left at home. . . . All are here for money . . . for which every sacrifice will be made. . . . In short, the sociable man is lost in the money-seeking, gold-hunting, selfish, acquisitive miser and conniving millionaire.

At what cost did that quest for wealth come? The knowledgeable goldfield physician, Dr. Jacob Stillman, estimated that one of every five miners died within six months of his arrival. That estimate may be conservative. Unaccounted for are those who died trying to reach the goldfields or traveling back home. An example is the saga of the Bute brothers from Guernsey County, Ohio. Nineteen-year-old C. D. Bute died January 30, 1851, at Grand Gulf, Mississippi, on his way home from California. His older brother died somewhere else, but a single tombstone commemorated them both.

The only statistical survey available related to causes of death comes from Sacramento, where 1,251 people died in 1851–1853. Of these, 58 percent succumbed to the following: fever, 252; dysentery and diarrhea, 237; the 1852 cholera outbreak, 102; and intemperance, exposure, and sundry accidents, 125. Close to another 10 percent died of "unknown" causes.

California, from seaport to mountain mining camp, had been converted into a "pest hole" within a year. The Argonauts may have seen California as an earthly paradise, but they managed to foul their nest. They blamed everyone and everything but themselves for despoiling the land. The wonder may be that more did not die. The outdoor life and the strenuous labor eventually contributed to the physical strength of the mining population.

By the 1860s improvements in transportation, the development of agriculture, and a more permanent population, in addition to better medical facilities and more highly trained physicians, led to a more healthful environment. The rapid decline of placer mining, replaced only in part by more permanent hard-rock and hydraulic mines and towns, assisted in the transformation. Even such a small matter as an increase in the number of cats and terriers to keep the rodent population (rat bites can cause fever, for example) under control made a contribution. The salubrious climate without doubt had a positive impact. Empathic convert Louise Clapp wrote to her sister that she left the mountains with sorrow: "[I have] gained an unwonted strength in what seemed to you such unfavorable surroundings." The "half-dying invalid" who boarded a ship to come west was "your *now* perfectly healthy sister."[13]

Clapp also provided the perfect epigram for the era of the forty-niners: "How oddly do life and death jostle each other in this strange world of ours! How nearly allied are smiles and tears!"

Notes

1. *California Star*, March 18, May 27, June 14, 1848. For a general overview, see Rodman Paul, *Mining Frontiers of the Far West 1848–1880* (New York: Holt, Rinehart, and Winston, 1963), 12–28, and *California Gold* (Lincoln: University of Nebraska Press, 1964), chapters 1–3.

2. E. Gould Buffum, *Six Months in the Gold Mines* (London: Richard Bentley, 1850), 68, 75–76, 93; Walter Colton, *Three Years in California* (New York: A. S. Barnes, 1850), 252; Richard A. Dwyer and Richard E. Lingenfelter, *The Songs of the Gold Rush* (Berkeley: University of California Press, 1964), 15; Jacques Moerenhout, *The Inside Story of the Gold Rush* (San Francisco: California Historical Society, 1935), 20–23; Ralph Andrist, "Gold," *American Heritage* (December 1962), 7; *California Star*, May 27, 1848.

3. *Placer Times*, April 28, June 23, August 11, 1849; Dwyer and Lingenfelter, *The Songs of the Gold Rush*, 71, 109.

4. Paul, *California Gold*, 31–33; William N. Johnson, *The Forty-Niners* (New York: Time-Life, 1974), 61–69; Andrist, "Gold," 10; Anthony J. Lorenz, "Scurvy in the Gold Rush," *Journal of the History of Medicine and Allied Sciences* (October 1957), 482.

5. Georgia Willis Read, "Diseases, Drugs, and Doctors on the Oregon-California Trail in the Gold-Rush Years," *Missouri Historical Review* (April 1944), 260, 263–267, 269–270; Merrill J. Mattes, *The Great Platte River Road* (Lincoln: Nebraska State Historical Society, 1969), 83–84, 85, 228; Mary Bailey diary, quoted in Sandra L. Myres, *Ho for California!* (San Marino: Henry E. Huntington Library, 1980), 59, 74, 85; George W. Groh, *Gold Fever* (New York: William Morrow, 1966), 115; Elizabeth Van Steenwyk, *Frontier Fever* (New York: Walker, 1995), 53; James E. Davis, ed., *Dreams to Dust* (Lincoln: University of Nebraska Press, 1989), 17, 99, 150; Andrist, "Gold," 11–12; John C. Gunn, *Gunn's Domestic Medicine* (Xenia, Ohio: J. H. Purdy, 1837), 265.

6. Edgerly W. Todd, ed., *A Doctor on the California Trail: The Diary of Dr. John Hudson Wyman* (Denver: Old West, 1971), 60; Read, "Diseases," 269–270; Lorenz, "Scurvy," 477, 480–481; Louise Amelia Clapp, *The Shirley Letters* (New York: Alfred A. Knopf, 1970 reprint), 198; John D. Unruh Jr., *The Plains Across* (Urbana: University of Illinois Press, 1979), 345–346; Mattes, *Great Platte River Road*, 81–83.

7. J. S. Holliday, *The World Rushed In* (New York: Simon and Schuster, 1981), 328, 493; Joseph Conlin, *Bacon, Beans, and Galantines* (Reno: University of Nevada Press, 1986), 87; Alonzo Delano, *Alonzo Delano's California Correspondence* (Sacramento: Sacramento Book Collectors Club, 1952), 30–31; Paul, *California Gold*, 86–87; Daniel Woods, *Sixteen Months at the Gold Diggings* (New York: Harper and Brothers, 1851), 102; Friedrich Gerstaecker, *California Gold Mines* (Oakland: Biobooks, 1946), 34.

8. Clapp, *Shirley Letters*, 131, 212; Frank Marryat, *Mountains and Molehills* (New York: Harper and Brothers, 1855), 233; Paul, *California Gold*, 87; J. D. Borth-

wick, "Three Years in California," *Hutchings' California Magazine* (December 1857), 275; Kenneth Johnson, ed., *The Gold Rush Letters of J.D.B. Stillman* (Palo Alto: Lewis Osborne, 1967), 58; Johnson, *Forty-Niners*, 104; Kenneth J. Carpenter, *History of Scurvy and Vitamin C* (New York: Cambridge University Press, 1986), 111; John Bauer, "The Health Factor in the Gold Rush Era," in John Caughey, ed., *Rushing for Gold* (Berkeley: University of California Press, 1949), 104.

9. Stillman cited in Johnson, ed., *Gold Rush Letters*, 38; John Ingalls, *California Letters of the Gold Rush Period* (Worcester, Mass.: American Antiquarian Society, 1938), 16; Buffum cited in Hubert H. Bancroft, *History of California* (San Francisco: History Company, 1888), v. 2, 231–232; Conlin, *Bacon*, 69; C. M. Sawtelle, "Pioneer Sketches," Bancroft Library manuscript; *Grass Valley Telegraph*, October 27, December 11, 1853, and January 19, 1854; James L. Tyson, *Diary of a Physician in California* (New York: D. Appleton, 1850), 79–80; Buffum, *Six Months*, 128–130; Carpenter, *History of Scurvy*, 111; Lorenz, "Scurvy," 487, 492, 495; Bauer, "Health Factor," 98–101; Groh, *Gold Fever*, 207, 215, 223; Swain cited in Holliday, *World Rushed*, 373; Henry Harris, *California's Medical Story* (San Francisco: Grabborn, 1932), 77–78.

10. Bancroft, *California*, v. 2, 237; Elizabeth Page, ed., *Wagons West* (New York: Farrar and Rinehart, 1930), 232, 260; Holliday, *World Rushed*, 372–373; Mattes, *Great Platte River Road*, 82–83; Groh, *Gold Fever*, 223; Van Steenwyk, *Frontier Fever*, 77; Read, "Diseases," 274; Charles E. Rosenberg, *The Care of Strangers* (New York: Basic, 1987), 90–93; Bauer, "Health Factor," 105–106; Marryat, *Mountains and Molehills*, 104.

11. *Placer Times*, May 2 and 12 and July 28, 1849; Holliday, *World Rushed*, 314, 373; Laurence I. Seidman, *The Fools of '49* (New York: Alfred A. Knopf, 1976), 134; Johnson, *Forty-Niners*, 104–105; Todd, ed., *Doctor on the California Trail*, 116; Dwyer and Lingenfelter, *Songs*, 136; Bancroft, *California*, v. 2, 232; Harris, *California's Medical Story*, 74–75; Gardiner cited in Dale L. Morgan, ed., *In Pursuit of the Golden Dream* (Stoughton, Mass.: Western Hemisphere, 1970), 225–226; Clapp, *Shirley Letters*, 4–5, 30–31, 87–88.

12. Leon Gottlieb, ed., *Gold Mining Surgeon* (Manhattan: Sunflower, 1985), 26–27; *Placer Times*, November 24, 1849; *Mountain Democrat*, June 17, 1854; Tyson, *Diary of a Physician*, 9; George Groh, "Doctors of the Frontier," *American Heritage* (April 1963), 90; Harris, *California's Medical Story*, 120, 125, 209; Bauer, "Health Factor," 107; Clapp, *Shirley Letters*, 43–47.

13. Holliday, *World Rushed*, 370, 521; Read, "Diseases," 276; Bauer, "Health Factor," 101–103, 106, 108; Groh, *Gold Fever*, 171, 174; Clapp, *Shirley Letters*, 39, 215.

2

"A Right to Go to Hell in His Own Way"

NEVADA, 1859–1900

By MID-1859 CALIFORNIA'S PLACER CAMPS had seen better days; most, in fact, had faded into oblivion. Californians were ready and eager to stampede to new discoveries. News drifted over the Sierra Nevadas during the summer about silver being discovered in what had been considered a placer mining backwater, the Washoe Range. Nobody knew that one of the world's great mining districts, the Comstock Lode, was making its debut.

Miners hied themselves to what became Gold Hill and Virginia City, which sat astride the Comstock Lode. This was hard-rock mining from the beginning, involving different techniques from those of California's early years. Hard-rock mining meant digging into the ground, which took skill, equipment, and financing not needed in most placer operations. Permanence, expanded urbanization, a new metal, bonanza wealth, technological mining problems, and financial concerns bestowed a different flavor and temperament on the Comstock.

Had it come into prominence at any other time, this discovery might have attracted national attention to this isolated, barren part of Utah Territory, soon to be Nevada Territory. Eighteen-fifty-nine, however, was no ordinary year. Earlier finds in Pike's Peak country dominated the headlines, overshadowing the Comstock everywhere except in California. Californians brought their experience, finances, and equipment to tackle a host of new problems along with the old.

In 1861–1863 Virginia City gained the national attention the country's most prosperous mining town deserved. Neighboring Gold Hill and Silver City, down Gold Canyon, lay in its shadow. These were not temporary placer camps—census takers in 1860 counted 2,244 residents in Virginia City and 600 and 594 in Gold Hill and Silver City, respectively. By midsummer of 1863 Virginia had mushroomed to a reported 15,000 citizens.

The Comstock boomed as no other district had before it. Glorious days were these, and their essence was captured by reporter Mark Twain:

> Virginia had grown to be the "livest" town, for its age and population, that America had ever produced. . . . Money was as plenty as dust; every individual considered himself wealthy, and a melancholy countenance was nowhere to be seen. . . . The sidewalks swarmed with people—to such an extent, indeed, that it was generally no easy matter to stem the human tide. The "flush times" were in magnificent flower.

Virginia City grew to be the "largest and most important town in the Territory," wrote J. Wells Kelly in his 1862 *Directory*. He might have expanded on that theme to say it had created and sustained the territory.[1]

The startling revelations motivated prospectors to scurry across Nevada, as more electrifying discoveries seemed to come with each new season in Aurora and Austin, to name but two. Nevada emerged during the Civil War years as America's most prolific mining region; its silver and gold underpinned the North during the war. Thus began a reign of mining dominance that extended forward for two decades. Although Colorado jumped to a faster start, its placer districts collapsed. In the public eye, Nevada could legitimately claim the number one ranking.

As befit the Comstock's grandest community, Virginia City evolved as the medical heart of the territory. Barely recovered from its birth pangs, the town had acquired nine doctors and one dentist, along with forty-two saloons, by 1860. The saloons reflected the hard-drinking inclinations of the Comstockers and foreshadowed serious medical problems. Virginia's two neighbors boasted seven doctors of their own. Add the drugstores and midwives to the medical menu and one finds an imposing array of medical choices for such a young community. The booming hard-rock present and future of this mining town had existed in no other town in California.

Physicians came to the rescue none too soon, because by June 1860 four people had died of typhoid fever and one each of inflammation of the bowels, cholera, childbirth, congestion of the brain, and mountain fever. The doctors confronted several conditions that had not been critical in California. An elevation of over 6,000 feet held inherent hazards, one of them being severe winters. Washoe zephyrs, those infamous fierce winds, gave rise to mental and physical anguish. Twain immortalized them as "the rolling billows of dust—hats, chickens and parasols sailing along in the remote heavens; blankets, tin signs, sage-brush and shingles a shade lower." And to a degree unknown before, problems of sanitation brought on by a rush of this magnitude bedeviled everybody. As one unidentified local correspondent wrote, "We have had a dismal time of it, but such are the hopes of men and the confidence in the mines that there has been but little complaint." That confidence overcame any health worries.

The miners called their camps "cities," but writer and mining reporter J. Ross Browne, visiting Virginia City in 1860, saw them from a different perspective: "Frame shanties, tents of canvas, of blankets, of brush, of potato sacks with empty whisky barrels for chimneys sat amid smoky hovels of mud and stone." At Gold Hill the miners, "like so many infatuated gophers," burrowed into the hills to live and work. The residents in both places, Browne noted, were "rough, muddy, unkempt and unwashed."[2] Physical improvements came soon, but sewers, better sanitation, and pure water were deferred by cost and time demands—formidable barriers to progress for people caught up in this unprecedented mining fervor.

Virginia City's potential for prosperity intrigued many, including physicians. A young doctor questioned Browne about Virginia City's prospects for setting up a practice. With a touch of the humor for which he became famous, Browne replied, "Doctors are already a drug in Washoe. Brandy, Whisky, and Gin are the only medicines taken." Lawyers swarmed to the town in even greater numbers, and he predicted "an abundance of litigation there before long." With that prediction Browne hit the mark, but he missed on the subject of doctors. They were an urban necessity, even though reliance on home remedies predominated.

During his visit Browne observed that despite "the number of physicians who had already hoisted their shingles," sickness still stalked Virginia City. Like many mining community visitors before and after, he concluded that illness could be attributed "chiefly to exposure and dissipation." Browne also blamed many ills on the water, "certainly the worst ever used by man." He continued, "Filtered through the Comstock Lead, it carried with it much of the plumbago, arsenic, copperas, and other poisonous minerals alleged to exist in that vein." He blamed the water for his own attack of stomach pain and "severe diarrhea." Even the mining-inured Browne had never endured such discomfort as this: "The complication of miseries which I now suffered was beyond all my calculations of the hardships of mining life."

The Comstockers concurred, but in the rush to riches, better water got short shrift. As Browne observed with a blend of humor and truth, the problem could be easily corrected by mixing "a spoonful of water in half a tumbler of whisky, and then [drinking] it."

Others blamed poor food for a variety of ills. This might have been true in the very early days, but the Comstock soon became famous for its fine restaurants and boardinghouses. Twain pointed to the altitude as a deterrent to good health. Built on the side of Mt. Davidson, the streets of Virginia City forced a climb that left one "panting and out of breath," even though one could descend them "like a house a-fire." Twain believed the rarefied atmosphere of so great an altitude forced "one's blood [to lie] near the surface always"; the humorist concluded that lofty residents lay only a pinprick away from disaster. It is accurate that the altitude caused breathing and respiratory difficulties, increased heart troubles, and exhaustion for the unacclimated newcomers. Ironically, by the 1890s that same "bracing" climate had metamorphosed into one nowhere to be found "more conducive to health and longevity."

The abandoned mine shafts and holes scattered all over the Comstock contributed to a multitude of accidents. Unilluminated nights took their toll on pedestrians, and the resulting accidents became legendary. Dan De Quille [William Wright] devoted an entire chapter to them in his book, and the *Territorial Enterprise* recounted them with alarming regularity. Pedestrians faced the same problem in Aurora, where the *Esmeralda Daily Union* (September 2, 1864) recommended that owners cover the holes with the "best material, well secured." Mining could be as dangerous and even deadly to nonparticipants as it was to those directly involved in it.[3]

While the Comstockers searched for and found silver, built towns, and attained fabled status, the Civil War was raging back in the states. The westerners followed its course with avid interest, and the bullion they produced helped pay the costs of the war. Less obvious—or appreciated—were the medical changes also taking place.

The Civil War years and the next two decades brought some needed changes to American medicine, and those changes reached the West very quickly. Westerners in the 1880s reviewed with horror the treatment they and their predecessors had received only a short time ago.

In the war itself disease proved more deadly than combat by a two-to-one ratio. The familiar killer diseases—dysentery and diarrhea, typhoid and malaria—stalked their prey. Among military doctors, as with doctors on the trail and in the mining communities, the importance of good water, sanitation, and a balanced diet were coming under scrutiny as possible factors in promoting good health. The primitive state of medicine had improved little since 1848. As a wartime surgeon general explained later, "The Civil War was fought at the end of the medical Middle Ages."

But the war stimulated significant innovation in medical treatment. Medical services proliferated and became professionalized. Doctors learned new techniques for amputation and the administration of anesthesia, largely because of their wide use in treating serious wounds. Many rural physicians evolved into operating surgeons. Civilians became involved through such agencies as the North's Sanitary Commission and made a long-range impact on medical history. Civil War scholar James McPherson concluded that the war fostered a "philosophy of scientific inquiry, hard-headed efficiency, and disciplined humanitarianism that became a hallmark of postwar philanthropy." The Sanitary Commission, for example, served as the model for the American Public Health Association. Founded in 1872, it played "an important role in the subsequent modernization of American medicine and public health."

The conspicuous participation of both northern and southern women in medical care was an important outgrowth of wartime exigencies. Their mental, emotional, and physical skills for nursing helped finally to overcome male prejudices. After the war upper-class women took up the cause as part of a larger women's reform movement. Their work as nurses advanced the status of the profession, a major achievement in U.S. medicine. Soon after the war, nursing schools began to be established, and their number grew to 432 by 1900. Some male doctors, threatened by the prospect of educated nurses, objected, but eventually physicians came to accept and rely on trained nurses. Nursing rapidly became a popular women's profession.[4]

Medical schools also proliferated; this initially caused the general medical situation to grow worse. The number of colleges increased from 90 in 1880 to 151 by 1900, "most of them inferior" diploma mills. Fortunately, the best schools upgraded their teaching methods and opened the way to the future. These changes came as part of the general reform of U.S. higher education that produced the modern university system. Medical schools introduced a more rigorous curriculum, emphasized "learning by doing," added new subjects, and lengthened terms to nine months; in the 1880s some adopted formal entrance requirements. The increase in the number of medical schools and the laxity of their standards, however, frequently frustrated the goal of advancing medical training.

The American Medical Association (founded in 1847) and the American Association of Medical Colleges (1890) passed numerous resolutions and standards concerning instruction, entrance requirements, and similar issues. In practice, the results proved minimal until after the turn of the twentieth century. The gradual improvement that did come was helped by articles (starting in 1894) in the *Journal of the American Medical Association* exposing fraudulent medical institutions.[5]

Medical research made some strides as well. The last three decades of the nineteenth century produced a "scientific revolution in medicine" that has been called the "triumph of modern medicine." Europe led the United States in that field, as it did in medical education. Americans traveled to Europe to obtain the best education, at least until Johns Hopkins Hospital and then Johns Hopkins Medical School opened (1893). The two (essentially a unit) became an integral part of medical education and pioneered innovative ideas and methods eventually disseminated throughout the nation. During this time Robert Koch and Louis Pasteur transformed microbiology into a science; their isolation of specific disease agents proved critical to preventive medicine. Joseph Lister advanced the idea of antiseptic surgery, and heightened awareness of the value of sanitary reform spread throughout the profession. Yet the bacteriological revolution was not fully accepted until the twentieth century.

The importance of preventive medicine became apparent. The causes of typhoid, bubonic plague, malaria, and eventually cholera and yellow fever were discovered, and mortality rates began to fall as the terrible scourges of the past began to disappear. The scientific revolution in medicine increased the importance of chemistry, bacteriology, and other subjects, which should have strengthened colleges' demands for a stronger general education. Sadly, it did not at the time.

Improvements in the use of anesthesia, thus decreasing the trauma of an operation for patient and doctor alike, and the revolution in diagnosis and in understanding the causes of infection significantly increased the patient's prospects for recovery. Even so, hospitals were considered places to avoid, and most operations took place at home or, if away from home, in a boardinghouse or hotel. Most Americans still viewed hospitals as places to go to die, not to get well, and they also bore the stigma of pauperism and pest holes. The surgeon preferred that two rooms be prepared, one for the operation and the other for recovery; spectators and concerned family and neighbors crowded around.

Americans made contributions to medicine in unexpected ways. The tremendous growth of railroads in the postwar era expanded doctors' territories and shortened the time needed to reach patients—and the time patients needed to come to them. The telephone accomplished much the same thing, although its real impact would not begin to be felt until the 1890s.

Before the new breed of doctor arrived, however, the prewar- and war-trained physicians—almost entirely male—dominated—carried the day. Diagnosis was assisted by the more prevalent use of the stethoscope, medical thermometer, and eventually, in the mid-1890s, the X ray. Incomes probably ranged from $1,000 to $1,500 a year, and especially in small towns and rural areas, a second occupation was necessary. Farming (difficult in the mining West) and running drugstores were popular adjuncts to the practice of medicine. To reduce expenses, the doctor's wife often served as receptionist, bookkeeper, and nurse. Specialists, particularly surgeons, and women physicians usually practiced in the larger cities, where the best hospitals and medical care could be found. Even back then Americans proved litigious, and the number of medical malpractice suits rose as the century advanced. Judgments in the hundreds of dollars before the war leaped to the low thousands after it. Rising medical expectations, increased materialism, antiprofessional sentiment, and without question the growth of the legal profession all contributed to the increase in suits and judgment sums. Americans increasingly blamed people and institutions for their personal misfortunes rather than fate or God, as they once had done.[6]

These changes eventually had an impact on the mining communities. One innovation that arrived more quickly than most was the increased use of the patent medicines so popular during the war. Many veterans carried their service-acquired diseases or war wounds, and they turned naturally to the "cures" that had served them well during their army days. Tragically, many of the cures included opiates, and the veterans marched home addicted—the "old soldiers' disease" as it became euphemistically named.

Impressive strides in advertising and journalism, which dated from Civil War days, brought ever more alluring patent medicine and miracle medical "gimcrackery" advertisements to everyone's doorstep. The nostrum and medical contraptions manufacturers, caught up in a highly competitive sales world, resorted to lavish advertising after the war. A popular ploy was to publish a testimonial about an astounding cure. Wrote G.W.T. from Virginia City, Nevada, regarding Pulvermacher's Electric Belts:

> I have worn the Belt and Suspensory for six weeks, and every symptom of the diseases is gone. The night losses stopped altogether two weeks after putting the appliance on, and the old vigor has returned. I feel better in health and spirits; and can do a good man's work in the mines without fatigue. . . . Several of the boys here were in my fix, and got cured by your belt and Suspensory.

Pulvermacher's costly gadgets supposedly cured nearly everything including lumbago, deafness, morphine habits, dyspepsia, and "lost manhood." The ads did not ignore women, their "marvelous belts being the greatest blessing ever vouchsafed to womankind."

Not only did the manufacturers distribute medical advice and praise for their own products, but they also disclosed to the layman the failings of their nemeses—doctors. Chief among doctors' failings, according to the medicine makers, was their inability to produce more effective remedies for illnesses than patent medicines. Said G.W.T., "I was troubled for many years, and got medicines from half a dozen doctors in 'Frisco that did me no good." The campaign succeeded. At the turn of the century Americans were spending over $74 million on patent medicines, and local newspapers reaped an advertising windfall.[7]

In Virginia City J. Ross Browne declared, "Quack pills, sirups, tonics, and rectifiers stare you in the face from every mud-bank, rock, post and corner . . . in cadaverous pictures of sick men, and astounding pictures of well men." Comstockers and others were also entertained for the next generation by medical shows. A "perfect Babel of cries and harangues" from peddlers, showmen, and quack doctors "on a torch-lighted city lot, in a gaudy tent or bedecked frame" building beckoned the gullible, the curious, and the ill of Pioche, Unionville, Mineral Hill, and places in between.

The electrical machine man made his pitch: "Who is the next gentleman who wishes to try the battery? It makes the old man feel young, and the young man feel strong. A quarter of a dollar places you in a position to have your nervous system electrified." He claimed the battery cured all diseases of the nervous system. The benefits of California Soap-root Tooth Powder lay in its instant ability to remove "all stains from the teeth and leave the breath pure and sweet." Hall's Sarsaparilla at one dollar a bottle (six for five dollars) promised: "No other remedy extant . . . will or does cure" rheumatism, gout, pimples on the face and body, spring fever, and indigestion and makes that "lazy liver" come alive. Virginia City newspaper man Alfred Doten frequented the shows. He noted in his diary on September 17, 1891, that the Pawnee Medicine Show was the "best I ever saw here," claiming that "bushels of Pawnee" medicines were sold.

"Real men" went to hear Prof. Compton lecture on "physical causes that lead to divorce, or the separation of husband and wife." Ladies were not allowed "under any circumstances." Prof. O. S. Fowler, the "greatest living phrenologist," lectured on such topics as "love, courtship and matrimony" and directed his attention to women: "for ladies only, female health and beauty restored." In private consultations he talked with "parties wishing to know all about themselves." Even Prof. Fowler would have had a difficult time competing with William M. Bird, "the hair restorer." He invented the Imperial Hair Restorative, which "speedily" restored new hair and imparted "new life and vigor to old hair." All together, these men promised to resolve most of the eternal physical and psychological ailments that confronted men and women. How could the medical profession compete?

Local doctors, state associations, and the American Medical Association tried to expose the "nostrum evil." The evil, however, would not go away until regular medical practices and doctors produced better results. It would take federal regulation to finally bring control to the "nostrum evil."

Nevada's mining community physicians did their best to provide such treatment, treating their patients with remedies that were at the same time older than the California gold rush and as new as the war. They most commonly countered diarrhea/dysentery with laxatives, Dover's powders, and opium, perhaps along with epsom salts or castor oil. They alleviated malarial fever with quinine and quieted the sufferer with opium. A typhoid patient's symptoms dictated his or her treatment. Doctors relieved abdominal pain with hot fomentations, blisters, and cupping (glass cups used to draw blood toward or through the skin); fevers called for cold compresses to the head and frequent spraying of the body with water. Patients swallowed small doses of turpentine to cure intestinal ulcers.[8]

As the doctors advised and treated, the Comstock's first boom came to an end, and the district descended into a period of "borrasca," as Comstockers termed the hard times. Fortunately, in the years before the "Big Bonanza" of the 1870s, other Nevada districts opened or prospered. Austin and the Reese River Mines, White Pine, Eureka, Candelaria, Tuscarora, Pioche, and scores of others drew the eager and adventurous hither and yon across the valleys and mountains. Nevada appeared to be a gold and silver treasure trove. Where the miners went, doctors usually followed.

The old story repeated itself—men and women endured cold, hunger, fatigue, and a host of inconveniences in their frenzied search for gold and silver. Nevada held a fatal attraction. Louise Palmer wrote about her husband and his contemporaries: "No man who has ever breathed the air of excitement and speculation of Nevada can live and be content in the quiet of his Eastern birthplace." Another observer concurred: "The contagious frenzy of the worshippers in the temple of the god with the shrine of silver . . . affects all who witness it." Over the next hill surely lay the "big strike" that would bring wealth and comfort "in a day."

Traveling to reach these new "bonanzas" proved trying enough. "Clouds of irritating and suffocating alkaline dust" greeted the rushers in the valleys between mountain ranges. Gnats and flies made life miserable in their season, water was always scarce, and the "oppressive and debilitating" heat of the desert took a physical toll on those who wandered about Nevada.

No matter where the migrants went, the same aggravations cropped up to vex them. In Austin the dust was reportedly "unbearable." One wag described an Austin bath as "composed of 2 inches of cold water in a big tub with a piece of brown soap, a napkin and $1.50." Mountain fever also dogged the Reese River rushers, as did "lung fever." Notwithstanding, the *Reese River Reveille* (June 3, 1863) noted that the town's first death (Nicholas Ferland, who ate a poisonous plant) did not tend "to destroy the pleasing opinion that this is the most healthful of all the mining regions east of the Pacific."

Austin soon had doctors, drugstores, and a hospital—the typical medical amenities of the era. The editor of the paper did come up with a novel reason for building a schoolhouse: "It would be far better for their [little boys' and girls'] health, too, to be under a kindly teacher rather than running at large in the sun."

The smelter and mining town of Eureka lay under a crown of black smoke, "redolent with fumes of lead, arsenic and other volatile elements." Boosters predicted "real prosperity" and a "bright future" as the soot and black dust rained down, giving the town a "somewhat somber aspect." Breathing the "smoky heavy metals" associated with the dense black smoke did not auger well for the residents.

Slightly farther east the White Pine district produced a host of medical complications during its short, frenzied existence. The elevation (8,000–9,000 feet) and "cruel winds" gave no quarter. Heart problems, pneumonia, influenza, and colds took their dreaded tolls of illness and death. The sometimes "fearfully severe" winters and cold, wet springs intensified rheumatism. The *White Pine News* (April 10, 1869) fought to reverse this image, claiming the stories of sickness and death exaggerated the actual circumstances. It and others blamed "exposure, neglect and carelessness" for many illnesses. An 1869 smallpox epidemic had nothing to do with the altitude; nor did a typhoid fever outbreak that summer. When all the "bustle and hurry, noise, excitement, and confusion" died away in 1870, White Pine vanished from the headlines. A visitor left behind a perfect epitaph: "land of toil and excitement, suffering, disease, fabulous and sudden wealth, disappointment, and death."[9]

Pioche took root in the southeastern corner of the state, far from its contemporaries. Its isolation did not protect it from the illness and disease brought by the rushers. The *Pioche Daily Record* (January 1, 1873) called pneumonia the "most destructive of all diseases here." Two pioneers, Obediah Brown and John Bibinger, had recently died of it. Trash sullied the landscape, prompting the newspaper's editor to write that when those "Washoe zephyrs wing their gentle passage down Main street the eyes of the passers are not only filled with dust, but paper, old socks, rags and straw flying round in the most admirable confusion." Local concern and city fathers eventually prompted improvements.

Pioche was well supplied with doctors, with six practicing physicians (including one accoucheur, or obstetrician) and a dentist in September 1872. At the county hospital, described as under "good management" and "kept scrupulously clean," the sixteen patients reportedly seemed headed toward recovery. Even so, Mrs. A. H. Doscher chose San Francisco as the place to give birth to her "bouncing boy." Families who could afford to leave often sought a lower elevation and a more diverse medical world. Nonetheless, Dr. William Rogers gained local fame for curing a man with a reported 100-foot tapeworm.[10]

There would be dozens of White Pines and Pioches before the mining fever ran its course in Nevada. Physicians eventually came to be symbols of a camp's importance. Tuscarora, for example, proudly boasted that "lawyers and doctors were well represented," a sure sign that it was "thriving." Physicians did their best to find a cure for everything, but too often their best efforts proved futile.

Virginia City's Mary Mathews chose to nurse her son Charley through an attack of scarlet fever during an epidemic: "I could not think of trusting his life in another person's hands." When urged by a neighbor to call a doctor because children "were dying all over the city," Mary expressed a deeply felt concern: "That is just why I do not get one; I am afraid they could not cure him." Charley survived. Rachel Haskell in Aurora treated everything that came her way herself. During the late winter 1867, she and her family suffered from headaches, croup, sore eyes, colds, and "soreness and weakness."

One of the popular volumes from the "vast treasury" of family information books, the *Golden Manual*, observed in 1891, "Probably as many lives have been saved by good nursing as by good doctors." An earlier home remedy book, *Dr. Chase's Recipes*, provided its readers with more medical information than they could ever use. The author, Alvin Chase, covered a multitude of symptoms and cures including soaking one's feet and drinking herb teas (catnip or mint) for headaches. He apparently believed strongly in teas, because he advocated a brew made from bayberry and hemlock bark, combined with ginger root and cayenne pepper cloves, to "cure drunkenness." He went on to stress that *your only safety is in keeping entirely away from places where intoxicating spirits are kept or sold.* He would have been appalled by one woman who, unsure of her husband's malady, prescribed "calomel, ipecacuanha, camphor, quinine, opodeldoc, paregoric, salts . . . and a few other trifles." She "piously" believed that by using a multiplicity of remedies, "some one of them would reach the right spot in his system."

Alexander Gow was convinced that many physical and mental problems were caused by "impure thoughts, vulgar language, vicious company, obscene books, and lascivious pictures." Nevadans, Californians, and others of the mining West surely stood in mortal danger! For them, however, the familiar mining camp adage made much more sense: "Every man has a right to go to hell in his own way."[11]

"Impure thoughts" probably troubled few Virginia Citians as they watched the Big Bonanza far surpass anything they had seen before. Impure water did worry them. Not until the mid-1870s did "our patient and long suffering citizens" get relief from water the *Territorial Enterprise* (June 6, 1873) described as "about as bad as it can be. It is muddy and has a bad taste." It also contained a host of minerals. Although some argued that women liked the arsenic "because it improved their complexion," which in small doses it did, and miners believed it "strengthened their lungs," the contaminated water continually fostered illness. Finally, in August 1873, an ingeniously engineered system brought water from the Sierras. Comstockers went "wild with joy," and a feeling of relief spread throughout the community. Fresh, pure water removed a source of trouble for local physicians.

The state's largest and most varied medical hospitals and best physicians (twenty-nine in 1878, for instance) continued to practice on the Comstock, contending with a variety of illnesses. Alfred Doten worked with several of the doctors. In his forty years of Comstock diaries, he discussed many of the medical matters with which they dealt. They appeared to fascinate him, even to the point that he assisted with operations. His entries ranged from little John Roark, who, with his dog, fell down a ninety-five-foot shaft and lived to recount his adventure, to an Irishman named Patrick, who survived an operation: "Cut off about 2 inches of his penis—the head all rotten with pox—awful sight—took about ½ hour."

Few patients suffered such traumas. Mrs. I. James fell off a "dilapidated sidewalk" in the dark, severely spraining an ankle. Catharine Curran suffered from intemperance. Charles Hall tried to commit suicide, but salt, mustard, and other antidotes kept him from crossing "the dark river." Mrs. Duffy became temporarily "deranged" after giving birth. Joe Nelson took to his bed with weak lungs, and Fred Hyde suffered a badly broken leg when his team ran away. These incidents were more typical, as the *Territorial Enterprise* chronicled Virginia City's illnesses and accidents.

In Nelson's case the doctors recommended a lower altitude nearer sea level, so he went to California. This was often the advice for similar diagnoses. "It is best to get over the mountains as soon as possible to where the air contains some 'nutriment,'" noted the January 30, 1873, issue of the *Enterprise*. Mrs. Duffy also moved to California to an asylum, where there was hope for her recovery. Doctors also sent patients to Nevada's hot springs. At least three—Steamboat, Carey's, and Genoa—were within easy traveling distance of the Comstock. They promised, among other things, relief from "rheumatic, cutaneous and scrofulous affections." Supplemented with hotels, vapor and mud baths, experienced physicians, and "proper medicines necessary for invalids," the springs became popular havens for the infirm.

Less popular recuperation stops were the City and Storey County Hospitals in Virginia City, two of the best in Nevada. Most people still chose to be treated at home because of hospitals' ongoing reputation. As evidence, only 20 of Storey County's 280 deaths in 1880 took place in a hospital. The three-story County Hospital, with separate departments for males and females, treated 5,262 patients from late 1865 through 1880. The five leading diseases and the number of individuals affected were venereal (731), rheumatism (587), chest and throat (566), fevers (499), and alcoholism (490). The 1880 county coroner's report listed pneumonia, mining accidents, consumption, and heart disease as the leading killers.

Pioche showed a similar pattern. In 1872 seventy-two people died in the community, only fifteen of the deaths occurring in the County Hospital.

Pneumonia, "delirium tremens," and "abdominal dropsy" were the most common causes.[12]

Almost totally absent were illnesses related to food deficiencies. The California tradition of a "yen for fancy eating" traveled to the Comstock and throughout Nevada. Mining engineer Louis Janin observed that the "eating [in Virginia City] was far superior to any I have seen out of San Francisco." The miners relished a good meal, and many ate regularly in boardinghouses and restaurants. Chinese cooks and restaurants were especially popular, in part because they were cheap, although "elegant meals were one way a rich man spent his riches." Few Americans routinely dined out in these years, but for miners doing so was a common practice.

Restaurants and businesses responded. Virginia City acquired a reputation for both "varied and excellent" cuisine. Comstockers could well afford the luxury. At a time in the mid-1880s when common laborers in the East earned $1.50 for a ten-hour or longer day (carpenters were paid $1.70 for nine hours), Comstock miners earned $4 for an eight-hour shift, carpenters $5, and engineers up to $8. Board ranged from $7 to $12 a week, shockingly high to easterners, but locals took the prices in stride.[13]

It is no mystery why Catharine Curran and the other alcoholics succumbed to the lure of drink. Temptation lurked everywhere. The 1880 census takers counted 100 saloons in Virginia City and Gold Hill plus six breweries. Other stores sold liquor, and alcohol constituted a large percentage of patent medicines as well. Sales of beer and whiskey amounted to an average of 15 gallons of beer and 5 gallons of liquor (chiefly whiskey) for every resident in the county. Roughly $900,000 was spent to quench the thirst of 20,000 people. Eliot Lord reported that Comstockers called 1880 a "dry year" in "comparison with 1876." It is no wonder that Alfred Doten recorded liquor-related fights or that Catharine died of alcoholism. Doctors could do little to alleviate the problem—temptations were too great, weaknesses too many, and the drinking tradition too widespread and legendary in the mining West.

Doctors' best efforts to cure their patients met with varying degrees of success. The leading causes of death at Storey County Hospital in 1880 were fevers (36), pneumonia (35), smallpox (31), lung disease (29), "mania-a-potu" (acute alcoholism; 27), and miscellaneous injuries (20). Patients who died of smallpox constituted 22 percent of deaths, dysentery/diarrhea 12 percent, paralysis 12 percent, miscellaneous injuries 8 percent, and fevers 7 percent. Some figures are suspect because hospital terminology used in defining diseases and causes of death was not always consistent.

Virginia City physicians were a conglomerate lot. Nevada passed a medical practice law in 1875 in an attempt to bring some order to the profession, but the best intentions became victims of spasmodic enforcement, and individualism reigned supreme.

Regardless of their credentials, most doctors made themselves available to patients for an hour each in the morning, afternoon, and evening. Several were willing to visit any part of the state for consultation or to perform surgeries. At least four physicians in the 1870s were homeopathic who administered a minute amount of drugs to produce symptoms similar to those of the disease, a "like cures like" philosophy. One used electricity to treat "all chronic miseries." "Doctress" Hoffmann, "Female Physician," promised to "cure all kinds of Female Complaints and Diseases of Children." Treatment would be "strictly confidential." She had competition from Dr. A. B. Spinney, who promised free consultation and was "naturally impressed with the delicacy of the subject."

Chinese physician Hop Lock published testimonies in the *Territorial Enterprise* from his U.S. patients. J. Thompson let the world know that Dr. Lock's skills had brought a "speedy cure" to his venereal disease. He "cheerfully" recommended him. Dr. Lock promised "successful treatment" of consumption, bronchitis, dyspepsia affection, sore eyes, and private diseases. Another Chinese physician and surgeon, Dr. Gin Hin, made a similar promise regarding curing private diseases at "reasonable" charges. Six Chinese doctors were practicing in Virginia City and one in Gold Hill in 1878.

The Chinese and their medical practices had been a part of mining since the days of the forty-niners. Often discriminated against and forced to live in "Chinatowns" on the outskirts of camps and towns, the Chinese persisted in the "nooks and corners" of the mining West. Blamed for much of the opium traffic, seen as harbingers of a district's decline, and vilified as "eaters of rats," they were nevertheless in great demand as cooks, launderers, wood choppers, and house servants. They brought parts of their culture with them, including medicine and physicians. Both Chinese and non-Chinese consulted them and followed their advice. The Asians maintained their own medical establishment, largely because they were unwilling to deal with the language barrier involved in consulting a "foreign" doctor, not to mention their strange medications and methods and higher fees.

Chinese medical practices were over a thousand years old, and they intrigued many Americans and Europeans, many of whom resorted to them in a desperate search for a cure after other physicians and remedies had failed. Acupuncture, massage, moxibustion (cone-shaped lumps of wormwood burned on the spot to be treated), traction, strange herbs, and even "magic" (talismans) were some of the treatments not available from more traditional sources. Typical Asian treatment for Comstockers and others involved the use of such plants as goldthread, watermelon, tarragon, and ginseng. The last constituted virtually a medical miracle, recommended as it was for a variety of ailments including asthma, depression, heart failure, menstrual disorder, impotence, and rheumatism. Diagnoses based on pulse reading, the condition of the tongue, or the moods or color of the patient were novel for non-Chinese patients.[14]

Chinese physicians recommended barberry, balloon flower, and acupuncture for toothaches. American dentists, enamored of their foot-pump drills and chloroform, used other methods. Dr. M. Holmes, who billed himself as "the pioneer of this state," guaranteed that all his procedures would be accomplished in a "careful and skillful manner." Practical businessmen as well as professionals, dentists during the borrasca of the 1860s advertised "prices reduced to suit the times." Nevadans, like most Americans, paid little attention to their teeth until something went wrong. Preventive dentistry remained several generations in the future.

Pioche's dentist, F. C. Nichols, came as close as anyone to practicing the preventive concept when he advertised in the *Ely Record* (September 8, 1872) "don't wait until they [teeth] ache." He recommended seeing him to "avoid sleepless nights, save your stock of patience and your teeth." Unfortunately, he did not describe the specifics of what he had in mind.

The state's mining prospects turned gloomy in the 1880s. The Comstock and other older districts declined, and no major new discoveries arose to take their place. Deep mining's costs and complications drained profits as low-grade ore replaced high-grade. The mining adage "it costs a mine to work a mine" became more fully understood and appreciated. Virginia City, Tuscarora, Eureka, Belmont, and other towns lost population, and many camps fell victim to abandonment.

As miners and their contemporaries moved on to more prosperous mining districts throughout the West, so did the medical establishment. For example, Virginia City's medical community had lost all but nine of its members by 1887. Those who departed left behind a more stable state and a core group of doctors and dentists to serve the needs of those who cast their fortunes with the Silver State.

Back in 1868, an unidentified Nevada correspondent to the *San Francisco Evening Bulletin* had reminisced about "the old days" and the modern times:

> The pioneer immigrants of 20 years ago endured hardship of which the immigrants of this year will know very little. If he fell sick, the misfortune was aggravated by exposure and the absence of all the comforts and appliances which increased the chances of recovery. The immigrants of 1868 will assume no such risks as did these pioneers. . . . There are cities, towns, schools, churches, highways, vineyards, orchards, and farms.

By 1869 the transcontinental railroad brought even more refinements. Nevada had come of age.

That same year a proud and pleased Elizabeth Palmer wrote in the *Overland Monthly*: "Have I succeeded in convincing you that times have changed here, since Ross Browne wrote, or Mark Twain taxed his brain for horrible and fictitious locals?" She believed women had caused the refinement and made the difference.[15]

The doctors and dentists who pioneered and practiced during these years also made a difference. Without them the residents of the mining communities would have had a far more difficult existence, and the quality of life would have been much lower. The 1890s found a declining state awaiting news of a new mother lode discovery to energize another rush. Over the next mountain, into the next valley—it had to be out there somewhere. The medical community would go too, whenever rumor became reality, just as it always had.

Notes

1. Eliot Lord, *Comstock Mining and Miners* (Berkeley: Howell-North, 1949 reprint), 96; Grand H. Smith, *The History of the Comstock Lode 1850–1920* (Reno: University of Nevada Bulletin, 1980 reprint), 28; Mark Twain, *Roughing It* (Hartford: American Publishing, 1872), 302–303; J. Kelly Wells, *First Directory of Nevada Territory* (Los Gatos, Calif.: Talisman, 1962 reprint), 107; Henry Degroot, *Sketches of the Washoe Silver Mines* (San Francisco: Hutchings and Rosenfield, 1860), 22.

2. Kelly, *First Directory*, 117–168, 180–184, 206–210; Lord, *Comstock*, 64, 94, 201; Myron Angel, *History of Nevada* (Oakland: Thompson and West, 1881), 76–77; Twain, *Roughing It*, 159; Dan De Quille [William Wright], *History of the Big Bonanza* (Hartford: American Publishing, 1877), 103, 107; Smith, *History of the Comstock*, 19–20; J. Ross Browne, "A Peep at Washoe," *Harper's Monthly Magazine* (January 1861), 153–154; Ronald M. James and Elizabeth James (eds.), *Comstock Women* (Reno: University of Nevada Press, 1998), chapters 1–2.

3. Browne, "Peep," 159–160, February 1861, 295; Twain, *Roughing It*, 304–305; *Nevada and Her Resources* (Carson City: State Printing Office, 1894), n.p.; De Quille, *Big Bonanza*, chapter 19; Charles H. Shinn, *The Story of the Mine* (New York: D. Appleton, 1898), 69; *Territorial Enterprise*, scattered issues, 1860s.

4. James M. McPherson, *Ordeal by Fire* (New York: Alfred A. Knopf, 1982), 383–390; *Medicine of the Civil War* (Washington, D.C.: Library of Congress, 1969), 3, 9; George Adams, *Doctors in Blue* (New York: H. Wolff, 1952), 227–229; Kenneth M. Ludmerer, *Learning to Heal: The Development of American Medical Education* (New York: Basic, 1985), 38–39, 47–51, 123; William G. Rothstein, *American Medical Schools and the Practice of Medicine* (New York: Oxford University Press, 1987), 85–86; John Heller, *American Medicine* (Urbana: University of Illinois Press, 1981), 204–225, 291–298; Paul Starr, *The Social Transformation of American Medicine* (New York: Basic, 1982), 154–156.

5. Martin Kaufman, *American Medical Education* (Westport, Conn.: Greenwood, 1976), 120, 121–124, 127–137; James G. Burrow, *AMA* (Baltimore: Johns Hopkins University Press, 1963), 8–14; Starr, *Social Transformation*, 102–108, 112–125.

6. Sources for this summary of medical developments are Starr, *Social Transformation*, 65, 69–70, 112, 115; Kaufman, *American Medical Education*, 120–121, 147–149, 154–155; Ludmerer, *Learning to Heal*, 19, 29–39, 63–64, 73, 93; Rothstein, *American Medical Schools*, 41–42, 67, 69–70, 73–75, 77–78, 89, 92–93; James M. Cassady, *Medicine in America* (Baltimore: Johns Hopkins University Press, 1991), 76–79, 87–91; Brian Inglis, *A History of Medicine* (Cleveland: World, 1965), 144–145, 152, 155, 157; Richard Malmsheimer, *"Doctors Only:" The Evolving Image of the American Physician* (New York: Greenwood, 1988), 28–29; Robert Karolevitz, *Doctors of the Old West* (Seattle: Superior, 1967), 65, 97, 113; Ward B. Studt et al., *Medicine in the Intermountain West* (Salt Lake City: Olympus, 1976), 44; Kenneth A. De Ville, *Medical Malpractice in Nineteenth-Century America* (New York: New York University Press, 1990), 25, 27, 64–65, 89, 115, 190, 227, 229.

7. Adams, *Doctors in Blue*, 229; James H. Young, *The Toadstool Millionaires* (Princeton: Princeton University Press, 1961), vii, 100, 110, 165–169, 170; Burrow, *AMA*, 71–74; Richard Dunlop, *Doctors of the American Frontier* (New York: Doubleday, 1965), 5–6; Starr, *Social Transformation*, 127–130; Adelaide Hechtlinger, *The Great Patent Medicine Era* (New York: Galahad, 1970), 11; David Armstrong and Elizabeth Armstrong, *The Great American Medicine Show* (New York: Prentice-Hall, 1991), 190–192.

8. J. Ross Browne, *A Peep at Washoe* (Balboa Island: Paisano, 1959 reprint), 188–190; De Quille, *Big Bonanza*, 393; *Reese River Reveille*, May 16, 1863; Walter Van Tilburg Clark, ed., *The Journals of Alfred Doten* (Reno: University of Nevada Press, 1973), v. 3, 1800, 1802; *Territorial Enterprise*, November 17, 1865, and January 4, 5, 15, 16, 1879; Armstrong and Armstrong, *Medical Show*, chapter 18; Adams, *Doctors in Blue*, 227–229.

9. Lord, *Comstock*, 64; Louise M. Palmer, "How We Live in Nevada," *Overland Monthly* (May 1869), 462; Albert Evans, "Up in the Po-Go-Nip," *Overland Monthly* (March 1869), 273, 278, 280; J. Ross Browne, *Reports of the Mineral Resources of the United States* (Washington, D.C.: Government Printing Office, 1869), 384; *Territorial Enterprise*, August 11, 1873, and June 21, 1874; Rossiter Raymond, *Mineral Resources of the States and Territories* (Washington, D.C.: Government Printing Office, 1869), 80, 92–93; J. Ross Browne, "The Reese River Country," *Harper's Monthly Magazine* (June 1866), 26–27, 36–38; Degroot, *Sketches*, 22; Angel, *History of Nevada*, 465; Oscar Lewis, *The Town That Died Laughing* (Boston: Little, Brown, 1955), 15; John J. Powell, *Nevada: The Land of Silver* (San Francisco: Bacon, 1876), 246–247; *Reese River Reveille*, June 3, 27, September 26, December 10, 1863; Turrentine W. Jackson, *Treasure Hill* (Tucson: University of Arizona Press, 1963), 52–54; Albert Evans, "Among the Clouds," *Overland Monthly* (July 1869), 66.

10. *Ely Record*, September 1, 4, 8, 1872; *Pioche Daily Record*, October 14, November 13, December 1, 1872, and January 1, 4, 1873.

11. *Carson Daily Appeal*, December 22, 1877; Mary McNair Mathews, *Ten Years in Nevada* (Buffalo: Baker, Jones, 1880), 43–44; Richard G. Lillard, "A Literate Woman in the Mines: The Diary of Rachel Haskell," *Mississippi Valley Historical Review* (June 1944), 85–86, 94–95, 97–98; *Golden Manual or the Royal Road*

to Success (Chicago: S. I. Bell, 1891), 351; Alvin Wood Chase, Dr. Chase's Recipes (Ann Arbor: Author, 1864), table of contents, 104, 140–141; Evans, "Up in," 276; Alexander M. Gow, Good Morals and Gentle Manners (New York: American Book, 1873), 53; Smith, History of the Comstock, 29.

12. De Quille, Big Bonanza, 221, 231–232, chapter 32; Territorial Enterprise, May 12, 1866, January 4, 10, 1872, January 30, June 6, August 11, 1873, June 20, September 9, 1874; Lord, Comstock, 323–332, 436–437, 440–441; Russell R. Elliott, History of Nevada (Lincoln: University of Nebraska Press, 1973), 137–138; Clark, ed., [Doten] Journals, v. 2, 869, 896–897, 913–914, 957, also vs. 1 and 3; Reese River Reveille, April 18–25, 1870; Powell, Nevada, 212–215; Angel, History of Nevada, 587; Pioche Daily Record, January 1, 1873.

13. Louis Janin to Mother, July 8, 1862, Louis Janin Papers, Huntington Library, San Marino, California; Joseph R. Conlin, Bacon, Beans, and Galantines (Reno: University of Nevada Press, 1986), 132, 167, 189, 193; Browne, Reports, 384; Lord, Comstock, 200–201.

14. Lord, Comstock, 377–378; Clark, ed., Journals, v. 2, 899; Wells Drury, An Editor on the Comstock Lode (New York: Farrar and Rinehart, 1936), 122; Territorial Enterprise, April 12, 1865, January 4, 1872, September 8, 12, 1874; De Quille, Big Bonanza, 383; Hubert Howe Bancroft, History of Nevada, Colorado, and Wyoming (San Francisco: History Company, 1890), 292; Thomas Chinn, A History of the Chinese in California (San Francisco: Chinese Historical Society of America, 1969), 78; Heinrich Wallnofer and Anna von Rottauscher, Chinese Folk Medicine (New York: Crown, 1965), 37, 50–61, 100, 112–114, 140–155; Pierre Huard and Ming Wong, Chinese Medicine (New York: McGraw-Hill, 1968), 30–35, 46–68, 151–154; Pioche Daily Record, December 4, 1872.

15. Wallnofer and Rottauscher, Chinese Folk Medicine, 56, 60, 138–139; J. Ross Browne, "The Walker River Country," Harper's Monthly Magazine (November 1865), 709; Territorial Enterprise, May 11, 1866, January 4, 1872; Evening Bulletin, quoted in Browne, Reports, 709; Palmer, "How We Live," 463.

3

"The Stench From Them Was Simply Fearful"

CALIFORNIA AND NEVADA IN THE NINETEENTH CENTURY

THE CALIFORNIA GOLD RUSH EXCITEMENT of 1848–1849 brought tens of thousands of new immigrants to the Pacific Coast seeking their often elusive destiny in hundreds of placer camps in the mother lode country. The work was tedious, their commitment to their new homes tenuous, and their knowledge of effective medicines and hygiene meager. In important respects their experiences paralleled those of the early Virginians who migrated to Jamestown confident that they would find a new Eldorado. While California provided greater opportunities than colonial Virginia, nonetheless most of those who had made the trek in 1849–1850 left disillusioned, died, or lingered awaiting word of another "bonanza."

As immigrants from the states and abroad flocked to the goldfields of California, American physicians complained bitterly about the current status of U.S. medical practice and training. Writing in 1851, Nathan Smith Davis described the preparation of western doctors. Estimating that "scarcely one-half" of those doctors had been either examined or licensed, he concluded that "every species of medical delusion and imposition is allowed to spring up and grow without legal restraint." Even in the Old Dominion he noted that almost a quarter of those practicing medicine had no formal training. He argued that, using newspaper advertisements as an indication of the prevalence of quackery, $1 million was likely spent annually on medicines "which at best do little harm and at worst are a positive injury."[1]

The experiences and complaints of the Argonauts confirmed the generally poor level of medical training and practice of the earliest doctors in the mining camps. Meanwhile, mining, milling, and smelting underwent steady and profound changes in technology and procedures that altered the medical risks workers faced. California and Nevada became transitional mining societies in the mid-nineteenth century. Both initially attracted prospectors and miners because they were precious metal mining regions; California began as the one of the world's distinctively rich placer regions.

The earliest miners employed the time-honored shovel and pan. The early Comstock boomers also "panned" for colors but found the region's pay dirt better suited to quartz mining. By the mid-1870s mining had changed dramatically; in twenty years prospectors had formed first partnerships and then workers' cooperatives that evolved into industrial enterprises with thousands of absentee stockholders. The mining also changed, as men now worked for wages and labored thousands of feet underground or employed "miraculous" hydraulic technology capable of altering landscapes and polluting entire streams.

The early placering in California initially offered age-old hazards, as miners worked with equipment that had been used for centuries. Working with pans, sluices, and arrastras, the forty-niners labored as men had in ancient and medieval times. Renaissance writer Georgius Agricola (1494–1555) systematically studied mining and medicine. His *De Re Metallica,* published posthumously in 1556, remained the standard treatise on mining and metallurgy until the mid-eighteenth century. The early Californians used apparatuses and strategies of mining Agricola analyzed and encountered medical problems he described. For example, he warned mine operators about damp, cold mines and their harmful consequences for workers' health. He noted the debilitating effects of dust in dry mines: "If dust has corrosive qualities, it eats away the lungs, and implants consumption in the body." He also reported that "cadmia [arsenical-cobalt] . . . eats away the feet of the workmen when they have become wet, and similarly their hands, and injures their lungs and eyes." He recommended that in cadmia mines workmen wear rawhide boots, arm-length gloves, and veils for their heads. He also identified bad air, carbon monoxide, and dangerous fumes as underground risks for laborers. His careful analysis of health problems associated with mining and metallurgy anticipated what twentieth-century industrial physicians would refer to as occupational diseases.[2]

Mining had inspired industrial and technological innovation since the introduction of gunpowder for blasting and the invention of the Cornish pump, which transformed English mining in the eighteenth century. In the American context two important changes fostered continued experimentation: precious metal mining rushes created mass migrations of expectant laborers, and the technical challenges of extracting ore in an era of scientific research and technological innovation transformed the character of mining. Rodman Paul quoted one forty-niner who asserted that men "from every country but Russia and Japan" engaged in an endless routine of "work, *work,* WORK! *Work or perish!*"[3]

While traditional placering had changed little over centuries, the Californians quickly engaged in organizational and technical experimentation, which produced companies of men who modified sluices into rockers and then into long toms. Constantly searching for more efficient ways to process large quantities of ore, they next exchanged the pan and rocker for the newfangled hydraulic flume and nozzle. By the early 1850s the peculiar richness of the placer deposits led to "coyoteing," the sinking of shafts into the subsurface gravel deposits of the ancient watercourses. Coyoteing was the transitional development wherein the Californians (especially Cornishmen with hard-rock mining experience) tunneled through gravel to reach the bedrock from which the placer deposits had been leached by the flowing streams. Although not yet lode mining, the coyote holes put men underground in an unstable and dangerous environment where shifts in gravel unexpectedly trapped or entombed miners. When the shrill cry of "cave-in" rang out, miners abandoned their own diggings and flocked to assist an imprisoned comrade. Minimally, these cave-ins produced cuts and bruises and more frequently caused internal injuries, which generally proved fatal in this era. Not until well after the Civil War did U.S. physicians begin to perform successful internal surgery, which required sterile procedures as well as an understanding of the relationships of internal organs or strategies for fusing injured bone and cartilage. Prior to the adoption of antiseptics, even external injuries often became infected, creating painful and sometimes crippling disabilities. The coyote shaft constituted an intermediate step between placering and quartz mining, but its hazards exposed miners to dangers more commonly associated with hard-rock or ore mining into bedrock.[4]

As the Californians mined the gravel deposits and then identified and began to work actual quartz veins in the vicinity of Grass Valley, they learned the rudimentary mechanics of timbering—using mine timbers to create tunnels and cribbing to hold soft ground in place. Subterranean mining also required attention to ventilation, which became an even more significant factor when true hard-rock mining operations extended hundreds and eventually thousands of feet beneath the surface.

As the Argonauts reached California in 1848 and 1849, their work at the mines immediately compounded their health problems. Often arriving sick and malnourished, the miners began the exasperating and tedious work of placering. Working year-round in or along cold mountain streams, the miners were susceptible to a host of job-related illnesses: colds, pneumonia, hypothermia, and influenza, to name but the most obvious. In the technical sense these were not occupational diseases as industrial poisoning or miners' consumption clearly would become, although they caused sickness and sapped the miners' strength and energy. As noted elsewhere, mid-century medical procedures and remedies were primitive by modern standards; physicians employed bloodletting and depended on unproven remedies such as calomel, citric acid, hartshorn, opium, whiskey, physicking pills, castor oil, rum, peppermint essence, laudanum, sulphur pills, morphine, and untold quantities of patent medicines. The illnesses did not respond to these remedies, and the physical characteristics (damp, cold, or wet) of labor in early placer mining made the laborers more vulnerable to these diseases.

Although many forty-niners abandoned the goldfields within a few years, those who stayed became part of an increasingly industrial workforce that retained a modicum of independence only by joining cooperative mining associations. The majority slipped into an industrial proletariat that worked for men with capital. Changes in technology or status kept these men working in the placer camps, although some would eventually find work in the lode mines of Grass Valley in Nevada County. As placering opportunities began to play out in the 1850s, Cornish immigrants began to develop the hard-rock or quartz mines first located in the Grass Valley and Nevada City region. The quartz mines held promise for longer-term development, but work in them required skilled miners, positions the Cornishmen quickly occupied.[5]

In his classic quantitative study of Grass Valley and Nevada City, Ralph Mann discovered that Grass Valley's hard-rock miners sustained more serious injuries than did their placering brethren in Nevada City. He reports that E. F. Bean of the Grass Valley *Gazette* concluded that approximately one debilitating mining accident occurred per day, a phenomenon confirmed by the large number of crippled men selling goods in both communities. The statistics showed a "much larger proportion of Grass Valley female heads of household worked or took in boarders than did their counterparts in Nevada City; likely more of the former were widows with dependent children." According to Mann the situation in Nevada County was so bad that the county hospital nearly folded because it aided poor, injured miners. Logically, these California miners adopted a method of cooperative support that had prevailed in Cornwall. Men contributed a portion of their monthly wages to an accident fund.[6]

California's quartz or hard-rock mining had stalled in the late 1850s because miners had reached the limits of their technological expertise. Two events brought substantial change in the next few years—the immigration of experienced foreign miners, especially Cornishmen, and the discovery of the Comstock Lode on the eastern side of the Sierra Nevada. The rush to Nevada's Comstock Lode in 1859 created an immediate decline in California, as the most ambitious and talented miners hiked off to the east in the round of continuing "rushes" that dominated the imaginations of miners for more than a century. The new bonanza demanded quartz mining technology from its earliest discovery. Here men necessarily burrowed into the earth and extracted ore from the fabulously rich ore bodies.[7]

The Comstock became the model U.S. mining community in the third quarter of the nineteenth century. Its silver mineralization proved fabulously rich, but more important, extracting the rich ore posed new problems for mining technology. Virginia City and Gold Hill were located above one of the continent's distinctive hydrothermal regions—a phenomenon that caused the Comstock mines to become intolerably hot and humid at greater depths. Additionally, the presence of the superheated water meant the mines were wet and thus subject to flooding at depth. The soft ground on the Comstock was the product of brittle quartz and swelling clay. Eliot Lord concluded that "nowhere can the crumbling rock be trusted to its own cohesion without a prop." The width and richness of the ore bodies prompted experimentation with new methods of timbering. Philip Diedersheimer resolved the timbering problem with his square-set cribs, which were precut on the surface and assembled into four-foot by six-foot squares underground. This innovation became the standard method of timbering on the Comstock and soon was employed around the world in mines with similar problems.[8]

The extraordinary richness of the Comstock mines and the capital investments of corporations created the world's deepest mines by the 1870s. Under the steady pressure of profits and the sometimes elusive search for continuation of the mineralization, the mines extended thousands of feet underground. In these halcyon days commentators and visitors came to remote Virginia City from around the world—it became one of the marvels of the era. Thousands of others arrived with more prosaic purposes, namely to wrestle the ore from these underground depths. At its peak of production in the 1870s and 1880s, Virginia City was the largest community in Nevada, but even in the 1860s it had become a legendary producer—a fact that prompted the Lincoln administration to endorse Nevada's statehood in 1864.

The community soon attracted an assortment of physicians and apothecaries who treated the injuries and illnesses of the mine and mill workers. James Galloway was a typical Comstock miner of the era. He began working in the mines in 1875 and spent eight years underground. He suffered from an assortment of injuries that began with a sore finger, which kept him from working for eight days in May 1875. In September he suffered from an illness that kept him at home after 101 straight shifts. Over the next several years he suffered from a painful boil on his leg, which he attributed to the heat underground. On another occasion he injured his hand in a pump rod. These were the injuries serious enough to mention, but his diary concluded on the day his shirtsleeve became entangled in an underground blower he was tending on the 2,700-foot level of the Union Mine. He died after directing coworkers to try to save his arm. Although the reports of his injuries and illness do not describe whether he visited Virginia City doctors, he might well have visited a physician for the sore finger, which was probably infected, and the boil. His final injury, had he survived, would have necessitated the treatment of a surgeon, as well as a prolonged convalescence, and would likely have left him a cripple without prospect of future work underground. By the 1870s and 1880s Galloway probably received competent medical treatment in Virginia City. Except for his fatal accident a later generation would have characterized his injuries as slight because they disabled men for less than twenty days.

Reporting on metal mine accidents in 1911, Albert H. Fay lumped as slight injuries cuts, sprains, mashed fingers, bruises, dirt in the eye, slight burns, the effects of powder smoke, and similar maladies. Serious injuries kept men from work for twenty or more days and included broken bones, severe cuts and bruises, loss of eyes, as well as injuries causing death or disfigurement. In 1867 Alfred Doten, newspaperman and diarist, reported that he watched as one of Virginia City's physicians chloroformed Mr. Small, a mine carpenter with a mangled middle finger, and removed the injured digit below the lowest knuckle. Small had injured himself two weeks earlier when he had accidentally fallen and smashed his finger between the ground and a heavy mine timber. The time lapse between injury and treatment placed the man at risk before he even sought competent medical assistance. Fearing gangrene and conscious that the digit was unlikely to heal, the physician demonstrated a knowledge of appropriate contemporary procedures as he first anesthetized the patient and then amputated the injured finger. Although Doten did not provide a follow-up diagnosis, the carpenter likely survived and was able to continue his work underground.[9]

As the Nevada and California mines extended to greater depth and produced greater quantities of ore, production demands prompted experimentation with improved haulage. The mine cage (underground elevator) was the first major breakthrough in equipment. Based on similar needs for haulage in industry and dependent upon the latest technologies employed in the construction and transportation industries, the cage became one of the marvels of the 1870s and 1880s. The earliest cages were open platforms running up and down the main shafts with men, ore, and equipment. The vast workforces, Diedersheimer's innovations in timbering, and the sheer volume of ore and waste rock extracted on the Comstock necessitated new haulage technology. The cages ascended and descended through mines customarily divided into hundred-foot levels, normally the amount of ground conveniently mined in underground blocks. The point at which the main shaft intersected the level became a station, where men and materials were on- or off-loaded from the cages. Dan De Quille [William Wright] reported that the stations were roughed in with boards and that they served as virtual closets for miscellaneous paraphernalia, from miners' hats and coats to mining equipment. He also reported that they were places for lounging and conversation as men arrived or departed from their work underground. Eventually suspended on wire cables attached to surface hoisting engines, the cages became an early source of underground accidents and injuries.

The hoisting engineers controlled the speed and operation of the cages from the surface. Communication underground depended upon a system of bells that connected the stations, cages, and hoisting engineer, who used gauges to determine the approximate depth of the moving cages. Although they were practitioners of an inexact science, experienced hoisting engineers could stop their cages precisely at any desired level. Lord described a group of miners awaiting descent into the Comstock mines:

> When a cage reached the surface the waiting men took their places silently on the iron gratings which divided its interior into compartments or "decks." Some gripped a round bar above their heads to secure their foot-hold, but most were content to cling to the close-packed bodies of their companions. On the warning stroke of a bell the laden cage dropped swiftly down the dark shaft, passing station after station with their flickering lights and busy sounds, until the appointed stopping-place was reached.[10]

Running cages caused an assortment of frequently debilitating, if not fatal, accidents to underground workers. Since neither the operators (located on the surface) nor the passengers could identify obstructions or persons protruding into the shaft, accidents were common in the early years. For example, Cornishman William Truscott, a forty-year-old miner, was killed in 1867 as he leaned over to pick up some tools, was struck by an ascending cage, and fell 400 feet to his death. A similar fate awaited John Sinnott, a miner, whom Lord reported was crushed between a cage and the bottom of the shaft of Savage Mine in 1869. Such deaths were grisly and occasionally senseless, as Henry H. Mason reported from Pevine, Nevada, in 1875. Describing men in Pevine as quarrelsome and often lubricated with "Frisco honey," he explained that "there have been several deaths caused by the men punching each other off the cages used in hoisting ore from the lower levels, say down 800 or 1000 feet and for lowering men in to the mine. . . . It is a frightful sight to see their boddies brought up on the cage with their brains beat out and all mangled to pieces." When cages were first introduced in the 1860s, they contained no supplementary safety equipment to stop a plunge to the bottom of the shaft if the hoisting cable broke. Of such vehicles William Wright concluded matter-of-factly that "there was no dodging when a cable parted. All who were on the cage must go to the bottom of the shaft."[11]

Although safety cages and improved steel hoisting wire had been installed by the 1870s, one commentator in 1894 still described cage accidents as one of the miner's "perils." Although occasional cage accidents might end happily, as when a Nevada miner was rescued after being stranded in a shaft for half an hour, the situations were often tragic, as when the hoisting engineer of the Consolidated Imperial overwound his cage and cast its occupants into the sheaves or spilled them out onto the shaft house floor, where all died. Eliot Lord and Comstock miner James Galloway described a similar accident in 1879 when a hoisting engineer in the Union Mine accelerated his cage when he intended to slow it. His error killed two miners and permanently injured six others, but the ninth "miraculously escaped unhurt by grabbing the bell rope with a desperate grasp."

Such accidents provided the earliest impetus for a primitive form of first aid as miners rushed to their companions and tried to render aid. Knowing little about care of the injured, men did their best to obtain assistance for survivors. Physicians trained in the third quarter of the nineteenth century were reluctant to operate on internal injuries because all wounds "suppurated," and internal surgery ordinarily resulted in death. An equally important deterrent was the physician's knowledge that nursing care was rarely available to individuals with severe injuries. The Virginia City Miners Union was the first to consider employing a physician who would render aid to the injured. Although the union failed to do so, this ideal of self-help led Comstock unions to provide death and accident insurance, as well as to create visitation committees that assisted sick and injured members.[12]

The cage and the square set were obvious responses to the magnitude of the ore deposits and to the increased depth of the mines on the Comstock. Both depended on the increased explosive power of dynamite, which posed new problems for the early miners. Marketed as "giant powder," the new and more powerful explosive depended on a stabilized form of nitroglycerin first introduced in California by Edwin Morse. The new explosive produced new gases that caused headaches and dizziness. In late April 1869 miners in Nevada City's Banner Mine quit work over the issue of dynamite and the single-jack hand drilling it permitted. Miners on the Comstock had also objected to the use of dynamite and single-jacking. The reasons for their concern were medical—men were subjected to new hazards in poorly ventilated mines and, simultaneously, ran greater risks when working alone in mine stopes and tunnels. Even more important for the Comstock experience, dynamite combined with cages and square sets to promote unimaginably deep mining.

By the early 1870s the major Comstock mines had gone below the 1,000-foot level. Over the next two decades these developments would change the character of mining throughout the West and around the world, but at the time they posed new problems for the Nevadans. Agricola had described the dangers posed by underground gases, but now men faced not only accumulated gases but also oppressive heat and pressure. Lord noted that the heat first became noticeable in 1871–1872. He reported that workers began to suffer from pulmonary and rheumatic disorders as they were transferred rapidly from the superheated depths to the surface, where temperatures could be 100 or more degrees cooler.

> Transferred in a moment from a torrid to a frigid zone, in the passage from the foot to the mouth of a mine shaft, they went out from the shaft-works sweating and often half clothed into the keen frosty atmosphere of the mountain slope. It was no wonder that many a man reached his home half choked by acute pneumonia and spitting blood. By heavy doses of quinine, ranging as high as 120 grains in the course of 24 hours, and the free use of stimulants, the acute attacks were generally relieved; but they often terminated fatally, for the miners drank liquors so freely when in health that the remedy of the stimulants did not produce its natural effect when they were suffering from pneumonia, and the physicians feared to administer liquor in extraordinary quantities, as the normal action of the liver and kidneys was already deranged by alcohol.

The severe problems caused by exposure to the rapid changes in temperature and pressure were soon reduced by the introduction of change rooms with showers and better ventilation provided by supplementary blowers and compressed air pumps. James Galloway continued to complain about colds, which he attributed to the temperature changes, but he avoided the more serious problems of pneumonia and an as yet undetected silicosis or miner's consumption, as men referred to it in the late nineteenth century.

Lord described the seriousness of the severe heat in his commentary on the Comstock. His descriptions of the underground depths of the Nevada mines explain both the obvious health hazards of the working environment and the related difficulties all mines posed in this era.

> By the dim light of their lanterns a dingy rock surface, braced by rotting props, is visible. The stenches of decaying vegetable matter, hot foul water, and human excretions intensify the effects of the heat. The men threw off their clothes at once. Only a light breech-cloth covers their hips, and thick-soled shoes protect their feet from the scorching rocks and steaming rills of water which trickle over the floor of the levels. Except for these coverings they toil naked, with heavy drops of sweat starting from every pore. . . . Yet, though naked, they can only work at some stopes for a few moments at a time, dipping their heads repeatedly under water-showers from conduit pipes, and frequently filling their

lungs with fresh air at the open ends of the blower-tubes. Then they are
forced to go back to stations where the ventilation is better and gain
strength for the renewal of their labor.

Here was a superheated, ill-ventilated, and contaminated environment
where men worked amid excrement and decay. In 1873 one drill hole at the
1,400-foot level of Crown Point Mine struck water so hot it cooked eggs.
Similarly, the effectiveness of proper ventilation cannot be underestimated,
as experiences at the 1,850-foot level of Bullion Mine demonstrated. As
the drift extended, temperatures rose until the working face ranged from
130–140 degrees Fahrenheit (F). Work at this depth and under these conditions was "painful and costly" until the level was connected to another
shaft, whereupon temperatures quickly fell to 100 degrees F.

Compensating for the heat and resultant dehydration became a major
cost associated with operating the Comstock deep mines. Again Lord proved
the careful chronicler of activities. Noting that in some stopes four miners
could not do the work of one under ordinary conditions, he described individual miners drinking 3 or more gallons of water per shift and consuming
95 pounds of ice. He concluded that the situation was so debilitating that
work would likely have stopped without the introduction of the newly
developed compressed air drills. The situation at the Savage Mine incline
in July 1877 is indicative of the health problems this work entailed.

> The temperature of the water as it issued from the rock was 157 Fahr.,
> and the incline filled with almost scalding vapor; picks could only be
> handled with gloves, and rags soaked in ice-water were wrapped about
> the iron drills. Men could only stand for a few minutes at a time near
> the hot fountain, and the work was carried on by successive relays.
> Here the men . . . were forced to breathe this suffocating vapor till they
> staggered forth from the station half blinded and bent by agonizing
> cramps. When the pain was so great that men began to rave or talk
> incoherently their companions would quickly take them up and carry
> them to the coolest place on the level, where they were subjected to
> vigorous rubbing on all parts of the body, but particularly on the pit of
> the stomach. When the so-called "stomach-knots" disappeared under
> the friendly hands the checked perspiration again began to flow, and
> the men regained their senses.

The hot, humid, oxygen-starved, and befouled air caused men to grow
dizzy. As men began work under such circumstances, they initially experienced "loss of strength, loss of appetite, and the inability to eat or retain
food." Although this situation was temporary, changes in appearance lasted
while the men worked there: "the flesh becomes plump and firm; the glands
secrete oil rapidly; the skin grows smooth and slippery to the touch, and
the complexion is clear, if somewhat sallow."[13]

Visitors to the Comstock mines invariably commented on the extreme temperatures. In September 1881 Eben E. Olcott visited the mines and explained their unique characteristics to his wife. He reported that underground temperatures ranged from 90 to 130 degrees F. at the 3,000-foot level of Yellow Jacket Mine. In specific parts of the mine temperatures reached 158 degrees F., with water temperatures of 160 or more. He explained that all visitors changed into "company" clothes before they descended into the mines. He wore loose trousers, a loose flannel blouse, woolen socks, and rubber boots and carried a rubber coat, which he donned as he returned to the surface. Like Wright and Lord, Olcott compared his experiences to what he imagined one would find in a "Russian bath" or sauna—streaming with perspiration. Although the ores were largely exhausted by the 1880s, Henry C. Morris and his friend Fred Wilder found conditions unchanged twenty years later. Like Olcott they stripped and changed into woolen suits, high shoes, heavy gloves, and waterproof hats before descending to the 2,200-foot level of the Consolidated Virginia Mine. He too commented on scalding hot water and "steam so dense it was uncomfortable to breathe: we were shown some of the levels and stopes and were particularly interested in the rest or cooling rooms, which had rows of benches with perforated tops and trough-like bottoms that were kept filled with ice to give the men a chance to recover from the scalding heat when the mine was producing." The extraordinary heat at depth affected other Nevada mines, as W. G. Flanders reported from Tonopah in 1912: "The mines are awfully hot I lost seven pounds the first two days I worked am afraid to get on the scales any more."

Normal working conditions on the Comstock were bad, and they compounded the medical problems when new men ignored the warnings of their more experienced companions. For example, Tom Brown, a Gould and Curry miner, fainted after working on the 1,900-foot level, and transportation to the surface did not immediately restore his senses. Although modern physicians would recognize these problems as ones caused by oxygen deprivation and dehydration, newcomers to these depths ignored their companions' warnings and literally worked until they died. Missteps or accidental falls caused men to be literally cooked alive. Miner John Exley died in 1877 when he fell into waist-deep water in the sump of Hale and Norcross Mine. Lord reported that "he was immediately plucked out, [but] the skin fell off his limbs from his knees down, and unremitting care could not save his life." A similar fate befell Michael Comerford, who rolled into the same sump and died trying to pull himself out by grasping the mine timbers overhead. According to Lord, rescuing a man from such a mishap was "a cruel service." William Jenkins fell into the sump of Julia Mine on February 5, 1879, and was immersed in 158 degrees F. water; "he was literally flayed alive and cried for death, though his sufferings were somewhat relieved by injections of morphine."

Given the time lapses between these accidents and the miners' receipt of proper medical attention, modern physicians would struggle to save life or limb. In the 1870s–1880s morphine was the most humane treatment Comstock doctors could provide. Lord attributed other deaths to the rapid transition from the heated depths to the surface, but the cause was as likely a too rapid ascent on a cage that carried men up thousands of feet in three minutes or less. Contemporary medical science associates symptoms of nausea and dizziness with too rapid decompression, such as the "bends," an affliction of divers. Although modern medicine recognizes the potential long-term consequences of such decompression, men on the skips often lost their grip on the cage and thus slipped between it and the shaft, which invariably resulted in dismemberment or death.[14]

Health problems stemming from work in the superheated depths plagued all who worked in the depths of the Comstock, but their gradual, incremental impact caused them to seem less serious than the disastrous mine fires that were the notorious tragedies of the Nevada mining communities. One late-nineteenth-century commentator concluded: "Fires in the confined spaces of mines are the most appalling calamities imaginable. An explosion is over in a moment, but the slow suffocation by gas and smoke is a lingering death of the most agonizing kind." The Comstock mines were particularly susceptible to mine fires because their underground workings were extensive, their use of timbering (especially with the square set) unprecedented, and the flammable conditions in the near-boiling depths vulnerable to any accidental provocation. The first serious conflagration on the Comstock began March 10, 1866, when fire broke out in the 260-foot level of Empire Mine. Although there were no reported injuries or fatalities, operations ceased for two days while miners fought the fire with water and underground bulkheads. Lord concluded that the fire was brought under control only after it had consumed all of the underground fuel. In October 1867 another fire broke out in Ophir Mine. Although quickly subdued by the frightened miners, the Empire and Ophir fires were ominous portents of worse disasters to follow.

The first of many truly disastrous fires on the Comstock occurred on April 7, 1869, at Crown Point Mine. Presumably ignited by a carelessly ignored burning candle, the fire spread unnoticed through the 800-foot level until "the burning timbers crumbled with a crash and a blast of hot air was sent through the shafts connecting the Crown Point and Yellow Jacket." Burning in the honeycombed, interconnected mines of the Comstock, the Crown Point fire killed thirty-four miners in three separate properties (twenty-three in the Crown Point, five in the Yellow Jacket, and six in the

Kentuck). The fire was discovered just as the shifts were changing; one group of men climbed aboard the Crown Point cage and was hoisted to safety, but the prompt relowering and second hoisting of the cage brought out only the three Bickle brothers. One suffocated before the cage surfaced, a second passed out and then was dismembered between the cage and shaft, and the third reached the surface, only to die from smoke inhalation. The other men trapped on the 700- and 800-foot levels perished in the smoke and gases. Alfred Doten reported that the fire fighting claimed at least one additional life. Lord claimed the fire released noxious underground gases that produced "a pain near the liver, next they were conscious of an oppression in the chest and a gradual filling of the lungs with some inert foreign fluid; then followed dizziness and sudden insensibility." Fire struck the Yellow Jacket again on September 20, 1873. Six were killed and many asphyxiated. Arthur Todd reconstructed the painful death of Cornishman William Johns, whose plaintive shrieks filled the mine for hours before he finally died of his burns.

On June 24, 1887, a major fire again broke out at the Comstock. This fire was discovered on the 1,500-foot level of the Gould and Curry Mine. When the alarm sounded, all but eleven men escaped, five on the 400-foot level and six on the 1,500. The bodies of the five men on the 400-foot level were found on the evening of June 24—all had been asphyxiated as they tried to escape through an old drainage tunnel. The others were not recovered for sixteen days and were badly decomposed when located and removed to the surface for burial. On Sunday, July 10, Alfred Doten and Frank Trezona went to "Conboie's undertaking shop" to see the victims. Doten confided in his journal that "the stench from them was simply fearful and I had to cover my nose and mouth with my handkerchief—Could not recognize one of them—Their clothes had been removed and all were of a dark brown color almost black—ham rind—as though they had been baked or roasted brown in an oven, the flesh being shriveled & dry."[15]

Physicians could do little for the fire victims. They had no capacity to treat victims of severe burns and could do little for persons suffering from asphyxiation except get them to fresh air. Although no Comstock doctors revealed how helpless they felt, their capacity to treat such victims was limited to ameliorating their suffering in death. They could dispense morphine to ease dying's discomforts, but its use often provided more reassurance for the grieving crowd than for the victim. In such situations the clergy were more important than the scientific healers. Lord described the desperation that accompanied the terrible Crown Point fire of 1869.

Father Manogue and other humane Catholic priests moved about among the people, consoling them with the hopes of a possible rescue, and bidding them trust in God, the strongest shield and deliverer. There were no wild cries or despairing shrieks. The children could not understand the peril, and the hearts of brave women break silently. The weaker minds were stunned by the sudden horror of the scene, and many women stood staring vacantly, with clenched hands and swaying bodies, while they waited untiringly through the long days for news of their loved ones.[16]

Between 1848 and the early 1880s, medical science had begun to abandon centuries-old treatments like bloodletting, but dramatic improvements in the treatment of injured men came in the twenty years that followed 1885. The U.S. Civil War provided physicians with ample opportunities to work with bodily injuries. The growing number of industrial accidents in construction, mining, milling, railroading, and factory work offered physicians continuing challenges. Yet physicians' limited knowledge about bacterial infections, coupled with dirty and unsanitary working conditions, meant that even the most superficial injuries could lead to gangrene, and serious injuries in remote underground workings ordinarily had advanced to shock before the victims had a chance to obtain medical treatment.

Notes

1. Nathan Smith Davis, *History of Medical Education and Institutions in the United States, From the First Settlement of the British Colonies to the Year 1850; With a Chapter on the Present Condition and Wants of the Profession, and the Means Necessary for Supplying Those Wants, and Elevating the Character and Extending the Usefulness of the Whole Profession* (Chicago: S. C. Griggs, 1851), 162–165; John S. Haller Jr., *American Medicine in Transition, 1840–1910* (Urbana: University of Illinois Press, 1981), 234–279.

2. Georgius Agricola, *De Re Metallica*, trans. from the first Latin edition of 1556 by Herbert Clark Hoover and Lou Henry Hoover (New York: Dover, 1950). Agricola discusses the mining practices and technology in Book 6, pp. 149–218, and comments on the dangers of the workplace at the end of the book, pp. 214–216.

3. Daniel B. Woods cited in Rodman W. Paul, *California Gold: The Beginning of Mining in the Far West* (Lincoln: University of Nebraska Press, 1965 reprint of 1947 edition), 88.

4. Ralph Mann, *After the Gold Rush: Society in Grass Valley and Nevada City, California, 1849–1870* (Stanford: Stanford University Press, 1982), 12; Paul, *California Gold*, 88, 147–150.

5. Mann, *Grass Valley and Nevada City*, 82.

6. Mann, *Grass Valley and Nevada City*, 182–183.

7. Rodman W. Paul, *Mining Frontiers of the Far West, 1848–1880* (New York: Holt, Rinehart, and Winston, 1963), 34–41, 56–64.

8. Eliot Lord, *Comstock Mining and Miners* (Berkeley: Howell-North, 1959 [1883]), 89–90, 401; Dan De Quille [William Wright], *The Big Bonanza* (London: Eyre and Spottinswoode, 1969 [1876]), 134–136; William Greever, *The Bonanza*

West: The Story of the Western Mining Rushes, 1848–1900 (Norman: University of Oklahoma Press, 1963), 114; and Paul, Mining Frontiers, 63–64. For an account of the magnitude of early cave-ins on the Comstock, see Alfred Doten, The Journals of Alfred Doten, 1849–1903, ed. Walter Van Tilburg Clark (Reno: University of Nevada Press, 1973), v. 2, 823–827 (3/5–11/1865), 956 (10/25/1867). "This morning a great cave occurred in the mines at Gold Hill— About 100 men were below but all escaped, only one or two got scratched a little—PM I went down there—The cave occurred in the Empire, Challenge, Imperial & other neighboring claims—about 200 feet of the Comstock ledge, where it had been worked out was supported by timers—caved for the depth of about 240 ft—On the surface about 6 acres had sunk, engine houses, buildings and all, some of it two or three feet in depth—ground filled with huge cracks and evidentally still sinking— . . . Workmen escaped mostly by Yellow Jacket shaft—when cave occurred the wind came up the shafts so as almost to blow roofs off hoisting houses—knocked men down in the mines—blew cars, cages, and timbers about" (823–824).

9.   Lord, Comstock Miners, 403; Louise M. Palmer, "How We Live in Nevada," Overland Monthly 2 (May 1869), 460; John Taylor Waldorf, A Kid on the Comstock: Reminiscences of a Virginia City Childhood, ed. Dolores Bryant Waldorf (Palo Alto: American West, 1970), 8; John Debo Galloway, Early Engineering Works Contributory to the Comstock (University of Nevada, Bulletin 41, no. 5, Geology and Mining Series), 21; John Bernard McGloin, "Patrick Manogue, Gold Miner and Bishop," Nevada Historical Society Quarterly 14 (Summer 1971), 28; Albert H. Fay, comp., "Metal-Mine Accidents in the United States in 1911" (U.S. Bureau of Mines, Technical Papers, 1913), 9; Doten, Journals, v. 2, 957.

10.   Wright, The Big Bonanza, 224, 231; Lord, Comstock Miners, 312–313.

11.   A. C. (Arthur Cecil) Todd, The Cornish Miner in America: The Contribution to the Mining History of the United States by Emigrant Cornish Miners—The Men Called Cousin Jacks (Glendale: Clark, 1967), 190; Lord, Comstock Miners, 402; Henry H. Mason to Sister, May 24, 1875, in Henry H. Mason Collection, Correspondence, Bancroft Library, University of California, Berkeley; Wright, Big Bonanza, 229–230.

12.   A. Williams Jr., "The Miner and His Perils," Chautauquan 18, 4 (January 1894), 429–432; Lord, Comstock Miners, 407; Galloway, Engineering Works, 16; Arthur E. Hertzler, The Horse and Buggy Doctor (Lincoln: University of Nebraska Press, 1950), 6–7; Alan Derickson, Workers' Health, Workers' Democracy: The Western Miners' Struggle, 1891–1925 (Ithaca: Cornell University Press, 1988), 70–73.

13.   Mann, Grass Valley and Nevada City, 183–193; Vernon H. Jensen, Heritage of Conflict: Labor Relations in the Nonferrous Metals Industry up to 1930 (New York: Greenwood, 1968 [1950]), 13, 16–17; Richard E. Lingenfelter, The Hardrock Miners: A History of the Mining Labor Movement in the American West, 1863–1893 (Berkeley: University of California Press, 1974), 13–16; Agricola, De Re Metallica, 215–216; Lord, Comstock Miners, 374, 389–396, 400–401; Wright, Big Bonanza, 225–226, 241–242, 248.

14. Eben E. Olcott to Pheme, Virginia City, September 9, 1881, in Eben E. Olcott Collection, Box 1, Correspondence 1881, American Heritage Center, University of Wyoming, Laramie; Henry C. Morris, *Desert Gold and Total Prospecting* (Washington, D.C.: n.p., 1955), 35–36, and Morris, *The Mining West at the Turn of the Century*, ed. C. S. Lewis (n.c.: n.p., 1962), 20; W. G. Flanders to Tom T. Lane, Tonopah, July 10, 1912, in Tom T. Lane Collection, Box 1, Bancroft Library, University of California, Berkeley; Lord, *Comstock Miners*, 398–400.

15. Williams, "Miner and His Perils," 432; Lord, *Comstock Miners*, 269–277; Doten, *Journals*, v. 2, 880 (3/11/1866), 1041–1046 (4/7–5/20/1869), 1209–1210 (9/20–22/1873), v. 3, 1672–1676 (6/24–7/10/1887). In 1869 Doten reported that the body of miner Martin Clooney was not recovered from the Crown Point shaft until May 20; Clooney was "only bones & clothes—identified by clothes & watch—The whole was bundled up together in a small box to bring it up—Flesh pretty much all gone—It had been in water so long that there was little or no smell" (v. 2, 1046). Doten also recorded the death of firefighter William H. Williams, who passed out from asphyxiation and fell to his death in the Yellow Jacket shaft (4/19/1869, 1043). Todd, *Cornish Miner*, 202.

16. Lord, *Comstock Miners*, 271.

4

"Brewing Sage Tea for Some Tenderfoot"
COLORADO, 1858–1900

"GOLD AT CHERRY CREEK." "A new gold fever may be predicted as plainly at hand." The *New York Times* on September 20, 1858, created an experience of deja vu for its readers; it appeared that history was repeating itself as they read their paper. It had been almost ten years to the month that news of the California gold discoveries had reached the East Coast.

The article went on to claim that the entire "eastern slope of the Rocky Mountains [is] richly treasured with gold." This news produced unusual excitement because Pike's Peak country lay barely over the horizon, only four or five weeks from the Missouri River. America and Americans geared up for their second great gold rush in a decade.

The golden Rockies exerted a strong pull, but the storm clouds of escalating sectional conflict, compounded by a lingering depression, also pushed the fifty-niners westward. In the expectant spring of 1859, around 100,000 fortune seekers loaded their wagons and launched the trek to the promised land filled with faith and mining mania but lacking experience. Despite the California experience, these migrants were medically ill prepared for their adventure, a fact that seemed not to concern them. The medical profession had not advanced much in the past decade either. The fifty-niners planned to go west for a season, make their fortune, and return home to a life they could never have achieved otherwise. Times change, dreams do not.

The Pike's Peak rush mirrored both the earlier California rush and the contemporary Comstock excitement. As a placer rush it was heralded as greater than the one of 1849; a poor man would have a second chance to make his fortune. This time around, however, the fifty-niner would not be worn down by the trip. Not only was the distance much shorter and less arduous for people and animals, but no cholera epidemic rode along as an uninvited guest.

Once again these people evidenced an impressive sense of history by preserving letters and keeping diaries. Twenty-eight-year-old Edwin Bowen came down with "gold fever." His diary, kept from La Salle, Illinois, to Gregory's diggings, records only one illness—a toothache and accompanying fever. A Denver doctor pulled the tooth for $2.50. A veteran of the California rush, E. N. Patterson of Oquawka, Illinois, was determined to try again, although illness had driven him home earlier. When approaching the mountains he wrote in a letter to his hometown newspaper, "I must reiterate the fact that we are all remarkably well—no one been ailing except one man and he is a physician—he had a 'shake' and we told him to heal himself." Patterson went on to describe how members of his party had "particularly benefitted by the trip in health and robustness." A similar report came from lawyer Charles Post: "The company are all in good health." Comments like these were rare in 1849–1850.

It should not be assumed that illness and trouble did not plague participants in the 1859 rush. The infamous Smoky Hill route invoked this comment from a *Rocky Mountain News* reporter on May 7, 1859: "Every day we meet men arriving from the States by the above route, most of them in a famishing condition." Once the would-be miners reached their destination, they rediscovered the adage that no one had ever worked so hard to get rich without working. Former schoolteacher William Dutt spoke for many when he observed a few years later that this was a "hard country and a hard life a man leads in it." If one made mining his business, he concluded, "sufferings, privations and the hardships of life, generally, are more often realized than the object for which they are endured."[1]

Like the forty-niners before them, these miners suffered from poor food, fleas, and the effects of cold-stream placering. Rheumatism was a common complaint, both then and in later years. The afflicted blamed working in the water, the dampness of mines, and the altitude for the condition. Some came down with Rocky Mountain fever, acquired from tick bites or the "old ague." If quinine was available, the ailment created no great alarm. Unsanitary living conditions in the mining camps precipitated the same outbreaks of "filth diseases" described earlier; both the 1849ers and the 1859ers trashed their sites with indifference. No lessons from California were brought by the forty-niners who moved to Pike's Peak country.

The fifty-niners, however, suffered from a mysterious disease they called "mountain fever," which struck in the late summer and early fall of 1859. Whether this was one disease or several remains unknown; regardless, it created a serious problem in the mountain districts. Humorist Artemus Ward wrote a vivid account of his two-week bout with it that left no one laughing. Returning east from an 1863–1864 lecture tour in California and Nevada, he reached Salt Lake City, where he took to his bed. A local doctor poured all kinds of "bitter stuff down my throat. . . . I had a lucid spell now and then. I lay there in this wild, boiling way." When he finally awoke with a clear head, Ward found himself "fearfully weak [and] frightfully thin." He ended his account with typical humor: "But by borrowing my agent's overcoat I succeeded in producing a shadow."

Newspaperman Henry Villard, writing in 1860, believed the fever was caused by "copious rains," which started in the last half of July; "this together with general exposure, scanty and ill-prepared food, the free use of bad water and worse whisky, produced a ravaging disease." He concluded that "mountain fever" had a "typhoid character." It "demanded many victims," he wrote, "and caused many more to abandon their work and seek the plains." Miners far from home, like thirty-five-year-old Albert Stephens from Missouri, died with their quest for riches unfulfilled.

Perhaps the mysterious ailment was some type of malarial fever the midwesterners had brought with them, activated by the stress of working outdoors under adverse conditions. An old saying could have applied to any midwestern state:

> Don't go to Michigan, that land of ills:
> The word means ague, fever and chills.

The symptoms Villard described sound much like ones found among sufferers in California and Nevada. The ailment may have been a variant of typhoid fever, as he thought (Ward, however, blamed "old-style typhus"). Indeed, it may not have existed as a distinct disease. "Mountain fever" did not reappear in epidemic form in Colorado, and it seems unlikely that its true nature will ever be known. William Byers, in his *Rocky Mountain News*, studiously avoided discussing the fever, apparently fearing Pike's Peak country had harvested enough bad publicity. Easterners viewed the region as a humbug in any case until the 1859 Gold Hill, Idaho Springs, and Gregory diggings discoveries became widely known.

Colorado's placering districts proved limited compared with California's. Only months intervened before miners began burrowing into the ground to follow the gold veins. Hard-rock mining dominated Colorado, and after the first year its experiences in many ways paralleled those of Nevada. Denver emerged as the medical center for the territory; by the fall of 1861 at least six physicians and surgeons and one dentist practiced there. Denver was not a mining community like Virginia City but served as a gateway and a supply and transshipment point. Central City provided the best medical services in Gilpin County, the major mining district, and by the fall of 1864 boasted two doctors, two dentists, and one surgeon/dentist. Once again the farther one prospected from these points, the farther one removed himself from medical facilities.

One major difference in the Pike's Peak region was the higher average altitude than that in California or Nevada. Denver stood a mile high, and all of the mountain camps and towns extended above that altitude—some to over 10,000 feet. Altitude had an impact on all who lived and worked in the mountains.

Dr. Irving Pollok, who arrived in 1860, reported that the symptoms he treated in people living above timberline were similar to those of lead poisoning—"heart acting languidly," nausea, sleeplessness, constipation, and pain in the small intestines. He firmly attributed the cause to altitude, ruling out lead poisoning or bad food and water. He studied particularly a group of people living in McNulty's Gulch, on the divide between the Arkansas and Blue Rivers. Not only the people were affected, but their "dogs and cats all died within three months." He concluded that it was "almost certain death for cats and dogs" to be carried to high altitudes. He advised his human patients to be careful: "I do not believe that you could make out to fight your way and earn a living while you are struggling for health."

Longtime Denver physician Arnold Stedman reported to the Territorial Medical Society in 1876 that persons of "ordinary health and flesh" usually lose weight with prolonged residency at high elevations. He also concluded that some suffer sleep disorders and recommended that people with "nervous temperaments" should not travel to these high areas, as they would likely suffer "nervous prostration." Stedman held out hope that the next generation would evolve with a constitution better adapted to the rigors of high altitudes.[2]

These early Coloradans actually suffered from what today is known as altitude sickness. Mining at 9,000 feet or more taxed one's physical system and could produce health problems that ranged from headaches, fatigue, and lightheadedness to pulmonary problems. Doctors in Colorado became well aware of the problems within a decade. In the 1870s mining reached the lofty elevations in Leadville and the San Juans, where some mines lay at or above 13,000 feet. Altitude-related illnesses became more prevalent as the mines moved higher up the slopes.

Coloradans ultimately came to view the altitude as a blessing. A pamphlet on Cripple Creek in the 1890s proclaimed that once an individual became acclimated, he or she would find "marked improvement of their nutrition" and a better "expenditure of nervous energy." A one-year residence in the community would "increase the chest two inches." The author, Dr. J. A. Whiting, advised his readers that it was essential they "get plenty of sleep"; he recommended eight to nine hours a night.

Altitude problems aside, mining continued through both the boom and the bust years. A milestone in Colorado's history had been reached earlier during the Civil War years. The conversion from placer to hard-rock mining had been completed, and Rocky Mountain rivals had arisen in Idaho and Montana. Then mining slumped, largely because of complications related to refractory ore and smelting. As a result, the future loomed less bright in 1865 than it had in 1861. To make matters worse, it became obvious that the transcontinental railroad would bypass the territory. Investors shied away after an 1863–1864 frenzy over Colorado mining stocks collapsed and left many easterners holding worthless shares, mines, and mills.

The years raced along, but attitudes seemed frozen in time. Like Californians, many Coloradans considered a visit to the doctor only as a last resort; home remedies provided all the care they needed or wanted. Doctors, well aware of their shortcomings, labored under the stigma that they caused pain. W. B. Mead, who opened a medical and dental office in Missouri City in Gilpin County, promised to perform painful operations in the most thorough manner yet "causing the very least possible amount of suffering." Mead came highly recommended, a skillful practitioner with "excellent tools." The combination of dentistry and medicine was not unusual, as seen earlier. In this day before toothbrushes and dental hygiene, Coloradan's mouths, like those of other Americans, often displayed dental disaster. Those who had no problems in the present almost certainly would in the future. Because of the pain often involved in a dental visit, that visit was frequently postponed. By the time a patient finally did come in for a visit, extraction might be the only alternative. General anesthesia rarely consisted of anything better than a strong shot of whiskey.

The challenge of eliminating pain and coming up with something new gave quacks abundant incentive. Dr. J. B. Young and his "medical and business clairvoyant," Miss Jackson, landed in Denver in February 1862. They promised, at the patient's leisure, to prescribe for every disease to which human flesh could fall heir. This would be done by "reformed principles independent of asking any questions" of the patient!

Doctors faced an economic struggle in the mining communities as mining ebbed and flowed. Dr. William Grafton, for example, found too few patients to maintain his practice and migrated from Nevada City to Central City before finally settling in Denver.

One obvious reason for his and other physicians' troubles is the fact that people coming to Colorado brought their own medicines with them. For example, Brown College chemistry professor Nathaniel Hill, who traveled west to examine some mining properties for eastern investors, wrote his wife that he had brought a "stock of medicines" including the following:

Five small bottles of brandy, 5 of whisky, none of which I expect to use; 24 small bottles of lemon juice . . . 1 bottle of concentrated extract of ginger; 1 bottle of cayenne, a pinch of which I put in the water every time I take a drink; a pot of senna in prunes; a bottle of Perry Davis' Pain killer. I had with me "Martin's Life Cordial." . . . I carry all these last articles in a little hand trunk or medicine chest.

Hill's precautions proved effective—the healthy professor eventually solved Colorado's smelting problems and became one of the state's leading mining men.

The precaution involving drinking water proved well-advised. Miner Samuel Leach wrote his brother from the evanescent Sterling City that "our chief difficulty in the mountains is [finding] pure drinking water." The situation was bad enough, he believed, that "most of the springs and streams are strongly mineral and some are not good at all, but very bitter and alkaline." Furthermore, the springs became easily contaminated, "and there is much fever and mountain sickness." Streams "polluted through mining operations" also wreaked havoc.

The stream conditions in Central City appalled a visitor from Michigan in 1878: "The water supply, once abundant and pure, is now utterly destroyed by the mining interests." Tragically, the nature of mining and its relationship to the communities generally prevented the resolution of pollution-caused health problems. Closing down the mines destroyed the economic pillar and ended the primary reason for the camps' existence.

Central City and Denver became embroiled in a nasty scrap over health issues in January 1863. When Central City's *Tri-Weekly Miners' Register* reported the prevalence of smallpox in Denver, Byers struck back, charging the report was "designed to injure Denver" by keeping people away. The *Register* argued that the *News* had claimed "smallpox is raging in Central." Through their reckless and thoughtless actions, both parties treated the subject in "a heartless way," judged the Central City editor. Each paper claimed no smallpox existed in its community. The intense urban rivalry forced scare tactics that did no credit to either newspaper.[3]

Contagious diseases generated apprehension no matter what the year. An outbreak of smallpox in Nevadaville in 1885 caused consternation throughout Gilpin County and in neighboring Idaho Springs and Georgetown. "Considerable indignation" arose when some locals tore down the red quarantine flags. Nevadaville believed itself unjustly accused, claiming only six cases had occurred in the entire county. A sigh of relief was heard when the crisis receded.[4]

As did Virginia City's, Colorado's newspapers published health tips for their readers. Black Hawk's *Daily Mining Journal* (October 17, 1864) advised them to reserve for hot weather the suggestion that salt "is inimical to bed bugs" because they "will not trail through it." To rid the house of them, the paper recommended washing floors, partitions, bedsteads, and the like with a solution of salt and water and filling "all cracks they frequent with salt." On August 17 that same year the paper featured an article on poisons and their antidotes. Byers, in his *News*, the territory's most influential newspaper, highlighted an essay on the "fourteen ways people get sick." Although the publication date was January 25, 1865, it sounded much like advice from a forty-niner. He warned against careless food preparation, "drinking poisonous whiskey," and neglecting washing and baths. His last admonishment, against "reading trashy and exciting literature," seemed irrelevant.

Reading trashy novels probably ran a poor last in Coloradans' concerns about illness. A home medical book or a knowledge of home remedies seemed a more comforting source for identifying problems and providing treatment. Home medicines were usually strong and foul tasting. The ever popular poultices and varieties of plasters were readily applied when deemed applicable. Patients suffered through them all and probably tried to convince themselves they felt better, if for no other reason than that the thought of a second treatment was abhorrent.

Rachel Levon, the mother of author Anne Ellis, practiced home medicine in several mining communities. From Silver Cliff to Querida and Bonanza, she treated family members and neighbors: "The first medicine was whiskey, then came quinine and camphor (this camphor prepared at home from gum and whiskey); then turpentine." As Ellis wrote, "One was pretty far gone when one or all of these did not bring him out of it!" Her mother believed in binding a chew of tobacco over a sore; "fresh cow manure was also considered good for this." For kidney problems she used Oregon grape root brewed with rock candy, with juniper and "a lot of whiskey" added to it. Babies with bowel trouble received "brown flour" or rose-root tea.

Coloradans treated their illnesses while continuing to search for gold and then silver. Success rewarded their efforts, and by the 1880s Colorado had become the number one mining state in the nation. It had achieved statehood in 1876, proudly accepting the nickname "The Centennial State." Doctors found that new responsibilities came with the first state laws the following year. They were, for instance, required to keep a registry of all births and deaths they "professionally attended" and to file a quarterly report. As "far as practicable," physicians were to report to the State Board of Health any "information bearing upon public health." Finally, county commissioners were authorized to establish a local board of health to regulate such things as public health and safety, nuisances, infectious diseases, and the causes of sickness. A physician, or any other person, who violated these regulations could be fined. Compliance and enforcement did not come quickly, but the free-wheeling days of the medical profession were ending.[5]

To correspond with the progress being made by Colorado in other fields, the medical profession organized the Colorado Medical Society. Its meetings and regulations contributed further to increased professionalism. Dentists followed suit, organizing the Colorado Dental Association in 1887.

Dentistry in Colorado evolved more slowly than medicine, just as it had in Nevada. Doctors at first practiced both professions until dentists began to arrive in greater numbers. Their experiences proved similar to those of their medical colleagues. For example, when Henry Rose went to Leadville in 1879, he could find no office space and so began practicing on the corner of Chestnut and Harrison, the town's busiest intersection. Working mostly at night using a kerosene lamp, Rose attracted much attention from passersby. Attempting to alleviate pain, dentists increasingly used anesthetics such as chloroform, ether, and nitrous oxide; they were effective, but inexperience in their use created more problems. Colorado's high elevation complicated the effects of anesthesia as a painkiller, and patients sometimes reacted in fascinating ways. Rose often drew a crowd to watch the show. But whiskey and other depressants made things even worse.

Twenty years later Waltus Watkins opened a dental practice at Amethyst, near Creede. He told his brothers about a problem doctors did not encounter: "A great many of these people want gold crowns and bridges, & some of them want gold crowns on front teeth for display. They ought not to be put there of course, but I am not here to regain lost health. I crown them when they want it done." Some dentists, like Watkins, preferred less flashy crowns in their patients' smiles. He dabbled in mining and complained, "If it hadn't been that I had to stay at office nearly all of the time I think I would have been shipping ore before now."[6]

New associations and a new state, with new mining camps and towns spreading throughout the mountains, opened opportunities for doctors, who continued to arrive close on the footsteps of the first miners. They encountered both old and new illnesses and ailments. The generally unhealthy condition of the communities had not changed since the 1860s.

Pneumonia, at these higher elevations, emerged as a major killer, lethal to even the strongest and healthiest residents. Leadville (10,150 feet above sea level), which created the greatest excitement during the 1870s and was the state's major silver district, proved an especially deadly site. This "wondrous town" burst on the scene in 1877, and by 1880 the census takers counted nearly 15,000 residents. The number of doctors jumped as rapidly, from two in February 1878 to a reported fifty by June 1879.

They were needed, if the headline "To Leadville and Death" gave evidence of anything more than journalistic bombast and envy. To be "universally regarded as an absolute death trap" did not enhance Leadville's reputation. Pneumonia, erysipelas, and heart disease, abetted by the altitude, threatened the rushers.

More truth lay in the sensational accusations than Leadville was willing to admit. The *Evening Chronicle* (February 12, 1879) bristled over the "unfavorable rumors." It did its best "to overcome the slanders which have gone abroad," yet even the editor had to admit the prevalence of deaths from pneumonia.

The winter of 1878–1879 had taken a terrible toll, although the actual number of deaths remains unknown. The coming of spring did not improve Leadville's air quality. Henry Moody wrote his wife in September 1879, "The dust here is fearful and what with the smoke from the furnaces . . . Leadville cannot be said to be healthy at present." The smelters, there and elsewhere, showered smoke that carried lead, arsenic, and other minerals, which the process released into the atmosphere. For people with upper respiratory problems, the atmosphere posed special dangers.[7]

It proved more dangerous than just respiratory problems. Moody put his finger on a problem that exacerbated all other illnesses—smelter smoke and lead poisoning. Because of its importance as a mining district, sixteen smelters at one time or another cascaded smoke over the city. On a bad day Leadvillites wallowed in smoke. Leadville's ores were "composed chiefly of carbonate of lead or sulphuret of lead"; as Samuel Emmons's classic 1880s study pointed out, "the quantity of lead completely lost in the atmosphere is sensibly twice as large" as that caught in the dust chambers.

Emmons also concluded "that owing to the peculiar nature of the Leadville ores and to the great altitude," the volatility of the lead compounds was increased. A person could not avoid breathing the smoke or walking in or stirring up the dust. The health impact could be immediate, or it might result in a latent illness ranging from severe stomach and intestinal problems to damage to the nervous system.[8]

Clouds of smoke swirled about all mining towns and camps that had smelters. Altitude and the surrounding topography made the problem worse. For example, Eureka, Nevada—also a lead/silver district sitting at a lower elevation and in a more open location—had fewer health problems from smoke than Leadville.

The smoky environment threatened everyone, but Leadvillites generally refused to acknowledge it. Three hundred people died of pneumonia in 1880, primarily because of, as a Leadville defender pointed out, "drunkenness and consequent exposure." Another Leadvillite concluded that the "reckless disregard of those presentations absolutely essential to the preservation of health in our climate" doomed many of his contemporaries. J. Ernest Meyers, ever an optimist, predicted that Leadville would become "the healthiest

mountain town in the country." Leadville, like every other mining community, was loath to criticize the industry that supported it.

One does not have to look far to find other causes for Leadville's un-
healthfuless: the elevation, poor housing, exhausting labor, extreme cold,
bad water, poor sanitation, and limited diets. For those predisposed to mental
illness, Leadville's excitement, excesses, and fluctuations in personal fortune
could bring them to the breaking point. Mary Hallock Foote recounted
such a case, which involved Englishman Hugh Price who had "stayed in
Leadville too long."[9]

Leadville, as the state's premier mining town, attracted some of the
best physicians and medical facilities. Smaller, less wealthy communities
were not so fortunate. Caribou, in Boulder County, inaugurated the silver
decade of the 1870s. The community relied on itinerant physicians until
its one resident doctor, William Mann, opened an office mid-decade. Mann
operated a mine along with his practice. In 1881, to ensure his permanent
presence, the miners agreed to withhold one dollar per month from each
man's wages for a retainer. When the fifty-seven-year-old Mann died in
1883, no one replaced him in this now declining camp. From that time on,
residents were required to travel several hours to Central City or Boulder
for medical attention or to endure the long wait for a summoned doctor to
arrive. Mann's presence, however, could not prevent a diphtheria epidemic
in the summer of 1879, which among its many victims killed three children
of Samuel Richards's family in a four-day period. This tragedy finally forced
the community to improve sanitary conditions. As the *Central City Register*
(August 8) noted sadly, reform came only after "several darlings had been
laid away in their last resting place."

For all its Victorian sentimentality, the article in the *Register* accurately
stated the facts—improvements in sanitary conditions or in the water supply did not become a priority until after a tragedy had occurred. Epidemics
were rare, however. Mann, like other doctors, typically treated injuries from
mining accidents, childhood diseases (such as mumps), la grippe (flu), and
pneumonia and delivered babies.

Preventable deaths, such as those of the three children, occurred
repeatedly throughout Colorado in these decades. Mining districts more
significant than Caribou had trouble attracting physicians. In the isolated
San Juans in 1880, for instance, among nearly two dozen mining communities only Rico, Silverton, Lake City, and Ouray had resident doctors. The
small camps coped the best they could, with the twin problems of time and
distance the vital considerations in any emergency.

Most towns and camps were reticent about discussing such matters.
Newspapers did not like to describe local outbreaks of sickness and disease
because of the poor image the stories portrayed to outsiders. No town liked

to admit either that it could not attract a doctor because of its small size. Some illnesses, such as pneumonia, were so common they did not deserve special attention.[10]

A sampling of the obituaries of individuals buried in the San Juan County cemetery from the 1870s to 1900 gives a good picture of the kinds of illnesses and accidents physicians dealt with. Mining mishaps, snow-slides, and exposure each accounted for 16 percent of deaths, followed by infant deaths, 11 percent; pneumonia, 8 percent; and heart disease, 7 percent. These percentages differ noticeably from those of Storey County Hospital in Nevada. One reason for this difference is the higher elevation of the rugged San Juans. The entire region, 4,800 square miles, averaged over 10,400 feet above sea level, the highest of any U.S. mining district. Alcoholism claimed two lives, but hidden among the twenty cases for which no cause was given were probably more examples, as well as venereal disease–related deaths.

By the time Cripple Creek burst on the scene in the early 1890s, many modern medical advances had reached Colorado. As the state's richest gold district, Cripple Creek could easily afford them. Doctors, even specialists, moved in quickly (at least twenty-two in 1899 alone), and both Cripple Creek and nearby Victor had hospitals. When Dr. J. A. Whiting wrote about the district's health in 1897, he pointed to the winter of 1895–1896 as the only unhealthy period. He blamed a pneumonia epidemic on familiar factors of overcrowding, poor sanitation, and lack of sleeping accommodations. Now, though, he had nothing but praise for the "perfectly pure and wholesome" water, dry atmosphere, sunny days, and warm, "very salubrious climate." In his estimation, Cripple Creek had "very little sickness." The past year had seen only 16 deaths out of 128 cases of pneumonia and 11 fatalities out of 127 victims of typhoid fever. This was certainly better, he claimed, than the 15–25 percent death rate in the eastern states.

Like Leadvillites before them, Cripple Creek residents bristled when the New York *World* condemned the town as the "deadliest spot on earth." The reporter claimed one had been far safer in the Union Army. Locals, not bothering to question the historical fallacy of that statement, immediately bombarded the paper with statistics and emotional letters. The tempest in the teapot soon died away.

Mabel Barbee Lee, who grew up in Cripple Creek, recalled a diphtheria epidemic there. Her mother credited her escape from it to a "heavy dose of physic." She also recounted how her parents dealt with her mother's being in a "family way." Before her baby brother appeared, Mabel was sent away for a "visit," only to return to find a new member of the family firmly en-sconced. Middle-class families liked to tell their children that the baby was delivered by the stork or found in a basket on the porch. Few in a mining community had the luxury of sending their children away temporarily. Lee remembered little ordinary illness among her family and friends.

Neither did Anne Ellis, who lost her husband in a mining accident. Her baby was sick briefly, and she became ill from overwork after her husband's death; in neither case did she feel the need for a physician.

In part, perhaps, as a counterbalance to "jealous" eastern propaganda, Colorado promoted itself as a health mecca. Newspapers, "puff" articles, pamphlets, and speakers repeatedly marveled at its "invigorating air," dry climate, altitude that increased the amount of "ozone and electricity," low humidity, and sunshine. According to booster Frank Fossett, Colorado was "the World's Sanitarium." The hot springs and mineral springs, which, according to their promoters and clients, could cure almost anything, came in for special praise. Abundantly blessed by the thermal areas scattered throughout the mountains, mining community residents readily availed themselves of their benefits.

Idaho Springs, one of the sites that had prompted the rush of 1859, boasted an "unequaled cure for rheumatism" in a "salubrious" location. Glenwood's hot springs reportedly cured "blood poisoning, rheumatism, catarrh and cutaneous diseases." Ouray's were "known" to relieve "chronic forms of gastric trouble" and to cure invalids of all sorts. Trimble Hot Springs near Durango specialized in healing rheumatism, skin and blood diseases, and "chronic difficulties of all kinds." The even more celebrated Manitou Springs promised visitors the "Fountain of Youth." Between the effects of the climate and the springs, those suffering from "asthma, throat and lung troubles, dyspepsia and general debility" could expect to be "permanently cured."

In their desperation and with exaggerated expectations, many paid little heed to Edwin Solly, who warned in his pamphlet on health resorts that the invalid "may find the road to health . . . often rough and uneven." Those comments aside, he went on to praise Colorado's health potential. Although they may not have fulfilled all the promises made, baths in the hot springs and mineral water treatments did do some good, at least temporarily, especially for the aches and pains related to hard work and increasing age.[11]

The miracles promised by the hot springs and mineral springs came in second to those of patent medicines, the continuing bane of the medical profession. Their proponents did not even blush over what they claimed their products could do that doctors could not. A few examples suffice: Plantation Bitters promised to be a "potent invigorant" to overcome that "languid, unrefreshed" feeling. Dr. Cook's wine of tar offered a "positive cure" for coughs and colds. The digestive organs and nervous system benefited from Dr. Harter's Iron tonic, and another (Burnett's Flavoring) claimed cocaine cured dandruff and promoted hair growth. The ads even used doctors to sell elixirs:

IT HAS BEEN DECIDED
By the best physicians in this country and Europe, that tobacco is an antiseptic—that is beneficial to health and promotive of long life.

The medical profession found it difficult to compete with such tactics. Georgetown's Dr. McDonald, an "eclectic" physician and surgeon, launched an advertising campaign of his own. He promised to use the latest "modes of treatment such as electricity, vacuum, atomizing, & medicated vapor baths." He promised all "chronic and acute diseases would be treated without the use of calomel or mercury." The patient "will feel as if [he or she has been] born again."

Few doctors' professional ethics would allow them to make such outrageous claims. Despite the advances in medical schools and course work, Colorado's physicians into the 1880s came mostly from the "old school." Josiah Hall, who practiced in Colorado for nearly fifty years, recalled that when he came in 1883, many of the doctors (he believed 85 percent) were "two-year men" who trained under another doctor and enrolled in two or three lecture series. The situation had changed by the turn of the century. Even at that late date, however, only a few of the larger mining towns had a woman physician.

One of the new breed of doctors, Charles Gardiner, wrote about how hard it was to start a mountain practice, with two other doctors in the camp where he settled (unnamed). Despite his knowledge of "up-to-date medicine," which his competitors lacked, they had "the knowledge of human nature and a business sense that gave success." He supplemented his income by performing dentistry and even delivering a calf—something he had not learned in school; also new to him were some of the illnesses he encountered such as snowblindness and "cow sickness." Dr. David Dougan waited twenty-nine days at Leadville in 1878 and was down to his last five dollars before his first patient walked into the office. A slow start proved to be a fast finish, as his income reached $12,000 that year. Young Detroit Medical College graduate, the previously quoted physician J. A. Whiting, found success when he treated a patient who subsequently made a mining fortune and hired him as a company doctor.

Being a mining community physician was difficult. Long hours, low pay, isolation, and dangerous sick calls took their toll. Gardiner, for example, told of a harrowing journey he made to a mine at nearly 14,000 feet. He survived snowslides, snowstorms, and a crawl along a wind-shipped cliff. Hall pointed out that hours of riding in a buggy contributed to painful sciatic rheumatism. Interestingly, horseback riders did not suffer the same affliction.

Some doctors succumbed to alcoholism, others to drugs. A few broke the law. A Silver Plume physician took out a huge amount of insurance on a house that mysteriously burned down; after collecting his money he skipped town, leaving his creditors holding an empty bag. One doctor in Cripple Creek defrauded an insurance company by faking a death, and a Central City doctor went on trial for a death following an abortion.[12]

When Colorado turned its calendar to the twentieth century, it had come a long way medically since 1859. Denver had emerged as a regional medical center, accessible to the rest of the state by railroad. Its hospitals and some of those in the mining towns utilized the latest medical procedures, and specialists were practicing throughout the state. The pioneers of 1859 could look back to a vanished age and ahead to one that promised medical miracles they would not have believed possible only a generation ago. Anne Ellis's mother typified early medical practice: "She was always brewing sage tea for some tenderfoot, who was getting 'climated.'" The Rocky Mountain region could call on skilled physicians and well-supplied hospitals to serve the needs of its citizens in the mining communities and elsewhere.[13]

Notes

1. Edwin A. Bowen Diary, May 22, 1859, Henry E. Huntington Library, San Marino, California; Patterson and Post cited in LeRoy R. Hafen, ed., *Overland Routes to the Gold Fields, 1859, From Contemporary Diaries* (Glendale: Arthur H. Clark, 1942), 33, 144; *Rocky Mountain News*, May 7, 1859; William Dutt Letters, June 7, 1862, Henry E. Huntington Library.

2. Robert H. Shikes, *Rocky Mountain Medicine* (Boulder: Johnson, 1986), 26–28, 29–31, 39–40; Elizabeth Van Steenwyk, *Frontier Fever* (New York: Walker, 1995), 41; Artemus Ward [Charles Browne], *The Complete Works of Artemus Ward* (New York: G. W. Dillingham, 1867), 210; Henry Villard, *Past and Present* (Princeton: Princeton University Press, 1932 reprint), 57–58; *Rocky Mountain News*, July 23, August 13, 1859; Thomas B. Hall, *Medicine on the Santa Fe Trail* (Dayton, Ohio: Morningside, 1971), 87–88; Samuel Leach to Brother, June 21, 1864, "Reminiscences," *The Trail* (November 1926), 20–21; Irving J. Pollok, "Report on Diseases Peculiar to High Altitudes," *Transactions of the Colorado Territorial Medical Society* (1872), 26–28, 30; *Transactions of the Colorado Territorial Medical Society* (1876), 55–56.

3. *The Cripple Creek Mining District* (Cripple Creek: Morning Times, 1897), 25–26; *Rocky Mountain News*, June 15, July 27, 1861, February 8, 1862, January 15, February 26, 1863; *Tri-Weekly Miners' Register*, January 12, 1863; *Miner's Register*, October 13, 1864; Nathaniel Hill to Wife, June 5, 1864, Colorado Historical Society, Denver, Colorado; Leach to Brother, June 21, 1864, "Reminiscences," 20; Sidney Glazer, ed., "A Michigan Correspondent in Colorado, 1878," *Colorado Magazine* (July 1960), 211.

4. *Rocky Mountain News*, March 14, 28, April 5, 1885.

5. Shikes, *Rocky Mountain Medicine*, 30, 35, 38; *General Laws of the State of Colorado* (Denver: Tribune Printing House, 1877), 703–712; Anne Ellis, *The Life of an Ordinary Woman* (Lincoln: University of Nebraska Press, 1980 reprint), 42–44.

6. Harvey Sethman, ed., *A Century of Colorado Medicine 1871–1971* (Denver: n.p., 1971); William A. Douglas, *History of Dentistry in Colorado* (Denver: Colorado State Dental Association, 1959), 1–17; *La Plata Miner*, July 4, 1882; Waltus Jewell Watkins, "A Frontier Dentist, 1898–1907," in Carl Ubbelohde et al., eds., *A Colorado Reader* (Boulder: Pruett, 1982), 183–184.

7. *Denver Tribune*, February 24, 1878; *Engineering and Mining Journal*, April 6, 1879; *Mining and Scientific Press*, April 5, 1879; *Leslie's Illustrated*, April 12, 1879, 87; *History of the Arkansas Valley* (Chicago: O. L. Baskin, 1881), 306–308; William B. Vickers, *History of the City of Denver* (Chicago: O. L. Baskin, 1880), 69; Henry Moody to Wife, September 21, 1879, Western Historical Collections, University of Colorado, Boulder; Rodman W. Paul, ed., *A Victorian Gentlewoman* (San Marino: Huntington Library, 1972), 203–204.

8. Samuel Emmons, *Geology and Mining Industry of Leadville, Colorado* (Washington, D.C.: Government Printing Office, 1886), 615–616, 625, 745–747; Edward Blair, *Leadville: Colorado's Magic City* (Boulder: Pruett, 1980), 94–104.

9. Paul, *Victorian Gentlewoman*, 204.

10. *Daily Register*, May 5, 1871; *Boulder News and Courier*, July 1, 1881, May 4, 1883; *Mining News*, December 31, 1884; *Colorado State Business Directory* (Denver: J. A. Blake, 1880), 124–126, 214–217; James Gibbons, *In the San Juan* (Chicago: Calumet Book and Engraving, 1898), 81.

11. Freda C. Peterson (com.), *The Story of Hillside Cemetery* (Oklahoma City: n.p., 1989), 1–307; Whiting cited in *Cripple Creek Mining District*, 25–27; Shikes, *Rocky Mountain Medicine*, 54–56; Whiting cited in Josiah N. Hull, *Tales of Pioneer Practice* (Denver: Carson, 1937), 127–128; Mabel Barbee Lee, *Cripple Creek Days* (Garden City: Doubleday, 1958), 25, 33–35; Ellis, *Life of an Ordinary Woman*, 202–210; Billy M. Jones, *Health-Seekers in the Southwest, 1817–1900* (Norman: University of Oklahoma Press, 1967), 89–90, 93; David Armstrong and Elizabeth Armstrong, *The Great American Medical Show* (New York: Prentice Hall, 1991), chapter 10; *Transactions of the Colorado Territorial Medical Society*, 15; *Glenwood Springs* (Denver: C. J. Kelly, 1883), 5–8; Charles Denison, *Rocky Mountain Health Resorts* (Boston: Riverside, 1881), 5, 12, 29, 34–39, 45; Frank Fossett, *Colorado* (New York: C. G. Crawford, 1880), 107–111; S. Edwin Solly, *Colorado for Invalids* (Colorado Springs: Gazette, 1880), 1–28; *Colorado Springs, Manitou and Colorado City Directory* (Colorado Springs: Tribe and Jefferay, 1879), 5, 8–9; *Rocky Mountain News*, July 1, 1868, February 11, 1874, January 16, 1880, August 9, 1881.

12. *Colorado Miner*, August 4, 1870, December 21, 1878; *Dolores News*, February 4, 1882; *Miners' Register*, July 31, 1869; Armstrong, *Medical Show*, chapter 17; *Rocky Mountain News*, November 8, 1884; *Colorado Miner*, October 10, 1874; Whiting quoted in Hall, *Tales of Pioneer Practice*, ix, 24, 82–83, 93, 117–118,

127–128; Charles F. Gardiner, *Doctor at Timberline* (Caldwell, Idaho: Caxton, 1938), 25–26, 28, 32–33, 35, 48–54; Frank Hall, *History of Colorado* (Chicago: Blakely, 1891), v. 3, 442; Dougan quoted in Shikes, *Rocky Mountain Medicine*, 48–49; *Daily Register*, May 9, 1871.
13. Ellis, *Life*, 45.

5

"The Mining Section Is Full of Men With But One or No Eye"

MEDICINE IN COLORADO'S MINES, NINETEENTH CENTURY

THE COLORADO FIFTY-NINERS encountered a mining environment similar in most respects to both the situation in California a decade earlier and contemporaneous developments on the Comstock in Nevada. Unlike California, the placering phase of Colorado development was short-lived. Within a year of the early Pike's Peak excitement Colorado miners were turning to lode mining with its characteristic underground work and coordinated workforce. Although some Coloradans continued to prospect in mountain streams for decades, the productive placering phase proved brief—in part because, as in California and elsewhere, such placering elicited an assortment of aches and pains. The uniformly high altitude, the cold snow-fed streams, and the often racing mountain creeks created risky diggings in the early days. Whatever placer process the men employed, they were cold, damp, and often exhausted by hard work—conditions that invariably contributed to a weakened body and consequently a high incidence of colds, influenza, and respiratory ailments.

Medical science could do little for these illnesses then and, interestingly, can do little more than treat the symptoms where prospectors continue to placer in modern times. Nineteenth-century commentators reported that the environmentally induced maladies became less frequent and debilitating as the miners became acclimated to their work and its strains on body and mind. As noted earlier with reference to the situation on the Comstock, the medical profession continued to employ the same nostrums and remedies in the early 1860s as it had in the 1850s. Although the nineteenth century was a time of extraordinary advance in the field of medical science, the rapid development of new theories and more effective medical training was still decades away when the Colorado excitement drew men and women westward in 1859–1860.

Americans were drawn westward as the country and its leaders witnessed the breakdown of the republican consensus. Although the Civil

War rent U.S. society as no other event before or since, its shocking and prolonged magnitude of human tragedy and suffering had unintentional beneficial effects on the advancement of medical practice and procedure in the United States. The extraordinary growth of the military population and the carnage that accompanied the four-year conflict provided an incomparable laboratory for medical experimentation. As surgeons struggled to repair battle injuries—severe wounds, shock, disfigurement, broken or lacerated limbs, bullet or shrapnel penetration—they began to improve their procedures and practices. Because infection killed tens of thousands who received battlefield surgery, the doctors learned to work quickly but, paradoxically, preceded by less than a decade Joseph Lister's seminal research linking antiseptic procedures to the reduction of secondary infection. These overworked physicians were appalled by the carnage they encountered. For miners and industrial workers generally, the advances in wartime medicine, coupled with Lister's insights, led directly to better and more innovative procedures for treating all traumatic injuries. The wartime creation of the Union's Sanitary Commission and the postwar publication of the Surgeon General's reports on battlefield medical and surgical practices during the conflict were major accomplishments in the history of American medicine.[1]

In particular, the Surgeon General's reports—which included both statistical reports on illnesses and injuries and abbreviated reports from field surgeons and physicians—constituted an important addition to the fields of military and general medicine. The number of military medical "regulars" (surgeons and assistant surgeons) jumped from a mere 100 at the beginning of the conflict to approximately 9,000 medical officers who served formally in the Union and Confederate Armies, as well as an indeterminate number of reserve surgeons who came to the battlefields to practice their medical skills. Since the 1860 census identified 55,055 physicians and 5,606 dentists in 1860 and 64,414 physicians and 7,988 dentists in 1870, approximately 12 to perhaps 20 percent of U.S. medical personnel served in the Union or Confederate Army or assisted with battlefield surgery during the four-year conflict. Some of these doctors found their way into the mining West while serving with the U.S. Army, and more followed the various rushes into the mining communities of the West. Although no one has determined precisely how many followed this route, historians have long known that many Civil War veterans drifted westward after the war. Physicians and dentists were unlikely an exception to these broader social trends.[2]

Military practitioners prescribed various forms of opium (laudanum, paregoric, or morphine) to "kill the pain" and employed ether and chloroform as anesthetics. Chloroform became the anesthetic of choice because it was not flammable, a trait that likely also appealed to mining camp surgeons who knew their clapboard communities could easily catch fire and burn to the ground. Widely prescribed during the war, opium, ether, and chloroform became the standard postwar medicines. Along with quinine, wonder drug of the mid-nineteenth century, these substances found their way into most physicians' bags, chests, or cabinets. Their wartime utility was so widely recognized that even the Union blockade proved ineffective in limiting their availability in most Confederate military and civilian medical facilities.[3]

The most common causes of underground mining accidents in the nineteenth and twentieth centuries were object or roof falls, individuals' falls, explosives, and machinery, including haulage systems. Furthermore, the conditions underground, where injuries normally occurred, were unsanitary in the extreme. In 1873 I. J. Baldwin went underground in Gilpin County's Bob Tail Mine tunnel. What he described was typical of underground work until well into the twentieth century: "It was a weird scene before me, the grim and sooty appearance of the men, the dim [candle] light cast on the rocky walls, the clink and jingle of drills and machinery, and the red glow and hissing of the [small steam] engine combined, reminded me forcibly of that region presided over by Pluto." In late-nineteenth-century Colorado, miners ordinarily ate their lunches at or near their work site, excreted waste underground, as there were neither portable commodes nor provision for underground hygiene, and worked amid animal offal. This situation facilitated the transmission of contagious diseases, but, more critically, the common accidental injuries to extremities, head, eye, or back occurred in singularly unsanitary conditions. The obvious parallels in both the types and severity of injuries with those encountered by wartime physicians are obvious.[4]

In the era before employee first-aid training, injured miners depended on coworkers to assist them from the putrid depths and back to the surface. If the injury resulted from falling rock or ceiling, miners ordinarily sustained upper body wounds, which were often severely infected before the victims reached the surface. Although the location of the injuries might vary when men fell or injured themselves in blasting, the consequences were normally the same. If a doctor were readily available, the men arrived with temporary bandages typically from workingmen's clothing. This temporary remedy to suppress bleeding or to cover an open wound often introduced the likelihood of secondary infection before the patient contacted the physician. In contrast, however, with the unprecedented pressure on health services war produced, the daily pattern of injuries in mines was ordinarily unique and isolated. The consequence was that doctors rarely moved from patient to patient in such haste that they had no time or inclination to cleanse their surgical tools. This situation dramatically reduced the incidence of those twin killers of Civil War fame: Streptococcus pyogenes and Staphylococcus aureus. Until the mid-1880s injured miners were treated without the benefit of antiseptic procedures, but the mining town physicians had likely cleaned their instruments since their last surgery.

Major procedural changes occurred after Ernst von Bergmann introduced steam sterilization in 1882 and after the turn of the twentieth century when enlightened doctors began to use rubber gloves to further reduce the introduction of bacterial infection. Tragically, such infections need not have occurred because since before the Civil War doctors often had satisfactory antiseptics at their disposal: alcohol, carbolic acid, iodine, bromine, mercuric chloride, acids, and sodium hypochlorite. Unfortunately, they had not discovered the antiseptic strategies that would have drastically reduced or even eliminated bacterial infection. Stewart Brooks explained this unfortunate state of affairs perfectly when he noted, "The best antiseptic must be applied *before*—not after."

When doctors encountered severe lacerations or compound fractures of limbs or digits, they customarily amputated the damaged area. Statistics gathered from Civil War experiences confirmed that amputation was most effective if performed within forty-eight hours of the injury or wound. During the Civil War, U.S. surgeons adopted two types of amputation that marked medical practice for decades to come: "guillotine," which sliced the flesh to the bone above the damaged area and then cut through the bone with a hacksaw, and "flap job," which cut the bone shorter than the surrounding skin and flesh, permitting a cosmetically better-looking stump. Civil War practitioners saw advantages in both procedures. Those with the guillotine amputation probably healed more rapidly because without knowledge of antiseptic procedures, the flap jobs trapped bacteria within the amputation wound.[5]

Coloradan John A. Hitching traveled widely in the mining region and remembered clearly the special problems faced and the peculiar injuries sustained by Rocky Mountain miners.

> Perhaps the worst feature of mining life is the constant liability to accidents; these are considered *extra hazardous* by life insurers, calling for double premiums, and if the insured handles dynamite, as most all gold miners do, they will not insure at all. . . . The mining section is full of men with but one or no eye, and with fingers missing, while hundreds are cut down in their prime, by twos and threes, every decade.

Ray Colwell had similar recollections of Colorado's Cripple Creek district, which opened in the 1890s. Almost seventy years later he recalled that "the ambulance and the death wagon were common sights" in the last of Colorado's great gold camps. More recent statistics (1922–1956) on work-injury frequency show mining to be between three and four times as dangerous as manufacturing and working on railroads. In nineteenth-century Colorado, when isolation, employee ignorance, and prevailing medical procedures and practices were combined, mining posed continuous serious health hazards.[6]

The sheer magnitude of opportunities for accidental or careless injuries in the Colorado mining industry stagger the imagination and must have confounded the overworked mining town physicians of the nineteenth century. In an occupation where careful attention to safety cost both time and money, mining and its practitioners were often inclined to take a shortcut that might save several shifts or even months. Hence, old workings frequently escaped careful inspection. Men often found them convenient sites for dumping or excreting. Tunnels and drifts in Colorado granite were no wider or higher than necessary. Ventilation of older workings often proved unsatisfactory, grades were often steep, and the floors of mining and tramming areas were cluttered with rocks and unstable debris. As electricity, compressed air, and water were introduced underground, the conduits ordinarily ran along the same floors and tunnels as did the ore cars and the working, walking miners. These situations invited accidents, especially where men performed hard manual labor over long shifts (commonly ten- or twelve-hour periods) in ill-lighted underground works.[7]

Corporate records and managers' correspondence illustrate again and again the ease with which a healthy miner became first an underground accident statistic and subsequently a physician's charge. Consider the case of Grant Anderson, a trammer (ore car pusher) in Leadville's Ibex Mine in 1899. On May 24 Anderson was pushing his car through a drift when he dropped his candle and stooped to pick it up. In this position he was run down by a second trammer, bent over in exertion from the weight of his own car. The report of the event was preserved by Kenneth L. Fahnestock, the company agent, who described the situation to its insurance agent, Thomas F. Daly. The correspondence itself confirms that miner Anderson sustained serious injuries, but surviving records give us no clue as to their extent or the treatment accorded him. By contrast, we know that Cornishman, or "Cousin Jack," Richard Pearce fell 116 feet at the Fisk Lode, dislocated both ankles, broke one leg near the hip, and tore so many muscles that his situation was feared irreparable. Pearce spend two years in a hospital recuperating and then went back into the mines in time to fall victim to a falling rock that dislocated all his bones between his toes and ankles. Pearce's tribulations were recounted in the *Rocky Mountain News* on January 20, 1875. Given our knowledge of medical practice at the time and the hazards of hospitalization, one must marvel that he ever returned to work after his first accident. By the light of the time, Pearce's physician was a miracle worker.[8]

Accidents involving explosives remained common underground throughout the nineteenth century. Central City's Cousin Jacks—John Wall, James Hambley, John Rolfe, and James Penpraze—were all seriously injured in explosions. Wall and Hambley sustained severe chest injuries when a Giant Powder (dynamite) cartridge exploded and blasted them with powder, rock, and sand. Rolfe apparently invited the inevitable disaster when he held a lit candle and smoked his pipe over a powder box in 1876; Rolfe sustained injuries to his left side—arm, thigh, eye, and cheek. His partner Penpraze was shot with copper shell.

Similarly, Alfred Castner King, Colorado's mining poet, abandoned mining for verse when a premature explosion on March 17, 1900, blinded him and left him unfit for work underground. King recalled an almost hopeless desperation that "slowly rallied" as he lay for months a patient in various hospitals. His poetic musings, probably begun while he yet enjoyed sight, form a testament to one of mining's victims—a representative man who struggled to understand why he now lived broken and alone. His poetry as it survives in Mountain Idylls and Other Poems is introspective, often fatalistic, contemplating broken love, illness, death, even suicide. In the tradition of Walt Whitman, King used verse to describe events and experiences of the common folk. He became obsessed with life's paradoxes: love and desolation, success and tragedy, scenic grandeur and blindness, hope and despair. In "Life's Undercurrent" he captures the desperation of the turn-of-the-century hospitals wherein he describes the lot of victims of fever, unremitting pain, cancer, paralysis, consumption. Yet it was his own fate, as with all who suffered permanent disability, he found most difficult to reconcile.

> Within the precincts of a hospital,
> I wandered in a sympathetic mood;
> Where face to face with wormwood and with gall,
> With wrecks of pain and stern vicissitude,
> The eye unused to human misery
> Might view life's undercurrent vividly.
>
> That day with fetters obdurate and fast,
> With chain of summer, winter, spring and fall,
> Is bounden to the dim receding past;
> Time o'er my life has spread a somber pall,
> With sightless eyes I grope and clutch the air,
> My lot is now the hardest lot to bear.

Eugene J. Trotter, another San Juan miner, responded with similar determination as he lost his sight and the use of one arm in a mining explosion. Refusing to enter Colorado's home for the blind, Trotter operated a newsstand at Colfax and Broadway in Denver and wrote a bitter, mystical, anti-Semitic tract entitled *The Forbidden Fruit and the Prodigal Son*, printed privately in 1919. These two miners-turned-"authors" sought to reconcile their world with their own tragic life experiences.[9]

The actual sequences of events that cost Alfred King and Eugene Trotter their sight have not survived, but Leadville's Kenneth Fahnestock recorded what happened in 1901 to Charles Bargler. While working in the No. 8 stope on the eighth level of Ibex Mine, Bargler was picking sulphide ore when a missed round exploded and threw him back "ten feet against a stull across the top of a raise into the #8 stope." Bargler suffered a broken thigh, severely lacerated face, and a lost eye. Twenty-three years earlier George-town miners Jacob Swartz and George Stark were severely injured when they drilled into a missed fire. Cecil Morgan described Swartz as "blown up" and Stark as "fearfully burnt." Often the victims died, as Robert Livermore remembered. Unintentionally underground during a funeral for two such victims, he remarked: "In one of the stopes I noticed a machine standing at a queer angle, and suddenly realized that I was at the spot of the accident. It didn't need the further grewsome evidence of blood and brains splashed on the rocks to send me out of that place in a hurry." Such accidents and injuries illustrate clearly the types of medical problems Colorado doctors encountered in the state's remote mining camps.[10]

Livermore himself experienced a potentially debilitating eye injury in 1904 when a piece of steel exploded from his drill and lodged in the exact center of his eye. As he remembered the accident, he reported that "fortunately, it didn't pierce the cornea, or I would have been minus one eye, but it gave me trouble enough. Continuing to fester and to blind me, it at last forced me to go to Denver, where a remaining fragment was extracted by magnet." Although conducted in an era of greater medical knowledge, Livermore's eye surgery must have been a delicate operation for his turn-of-the-century specialist. The normality of such occurrences was reaffirmed by Fahnestock, who reported that miners Porkorney, Nelson, Astleeford, Gronick, and Cortellini all sustained injuries when their picks struck rock or steel and cast the percussion fragments into their eyes. Fahnestock explained to Thomas F. Daly that "a large percentage of the minor accidents in our mine are from this same cause, and while there may seem to be a great many of them I can see no way to avoid it."[11]

By the turn of the twentieth century Colorado mine owners and operators were required to file an annual accident report with the commissioner of mines. Responding to these new requirements, Fahnestock reported that between January 1, 1899, and January 1, 1900, Leadville's Ibex employed an average of 268 men underground and another 111 aboveground. During that year Ibex workers had completed 91,793 underground and 34,831 aboveground shifts. In the twelve-month period 3 accidents had ended in fatalities; there had been 122 nonfatal underground accidents, 41 nonfatal surface accidents, and 9 nonfatal injuries en route to work. Using the Ibex average workforce-size figures, Ibex miners worked approximately 343 shifts per year, while the surface workers completed approximately 314 shifts. This means the Ibex averaged a serious accident about every 2.75 shifts, with 3 fatalities during a work year. This human carnage kept the community physicians and Leadville's St. Vincent's Hospital busy. The seriousness of the accidents was compounded by the still primitive state of first-aid training, which effectively denied the injured prompt on-site attention to their wounds.[12]

The tragedy of those recurrent symbols—ambulance and hearse—is given dramatic representation in the sorrowful entreaty of Chicago's Anna Feageans to John F. Campion, Colorado mine owner and operator. Anna's son "Fea" had died in Cripple Creek's Henry Adney Mine on July 17, 1905—the victim, as she explained to Campion, "I am told through poor management of the mine." Like thousands of other mothers and widows, she bemoaned the loss of her beloved son: "I have worked all his life so hard, to prepare him to take his place as a man among men and just when I seemed to of reached the place in life to see him take up the duties which he was so anxious to relieve me of, I get that awful news that he is gone, gone out of my life only in the flesh for I know that he is with me always."

Similar situations recurred again and again in Colorado's mines. Leadville's John O'Hara broke his back in Mary Murphy Mine and was taken to Denver's St. Joseph's Hospital, where he lay dying in late December 1900. Three years later Patrick Peterson sustained permanent injury that took him first to Leadville's St. Vincent's Hospital and then to St. Joseph's Hospital. Although he won an injury settlement of $2,250, Peterson's expenses and invalid status soon left him destitute. Nearly broke by mid-August 1903, Patrick was unable to pay his bills and likely became a ward of the county.[13]

The problems posed by mining created injuries that were notoriously disfiguring. For example, in 1889 the wife of Aspen mining engineer Hal Sayre reported that one of the miners at Compromise Mine had an accident that nearly sawed off his leg. The man's condition required amputation the following day and left him an invalid father of five young children. Less dramatically, Leadville's Edward Cotter injured his back when he slipped while lifting a heavy rock; R. Walsey did the same thing while "lifting heavy timbers." Injuries underground posed serious dilemmas for those charged with aiding their coworkers. For example, Ibex Mining Company employee Pat Kelley was injured when a man-cage crashed into the No. 10 station in the mine. Unlike his two companions who were simply shaken up, Kelley was seriously injured. Since the Ibex company physician was a local doctor on retainer, the Ibex workers loaded Kelley onto a mattress and carried him to town. Although the nature of Kelley's injury passed unnoticed into history, the visual image of several men struggling to carry an injured colleague into town would outrage modern sensibilities about the need to provide both trained personnel and proper equipment.

Once again Fahnestock reported that Irishman James A. Sullivan was killed on September 3, 1898, when he was struck by a cage running in the Ibex Mine's No. 5 shaft. Hearing the approach of the hoisting cage, Sullivan stepped into the path of the descending cage. He was killed instantly and qualified for a death benefit because he had paid the Ibex Mine's insurance premiums. These injuries had serious consequences for the miners, but even the regular work routine could prove debilitating. For example, Frank Crampton remembered that mucking "put blisters on my hands until they were raw and muscle pains in every part of my body that kept me from sleeping, but under expert teaching these tortures were soon over." Crampton described single jacking in narrow spaces as equally unsatisfactory. He concluded that "in narrow stopes there was hardly enough room to swing even a single jack upward without wearing the skin from the striking arm by scraping it against the Walls."[14] Although calluses formed in time, the innumerable opportunities for scrapes and bruises in this environment undoubtedly contributed to infections and minor health ailments.

Falling objects proved especially troubling to Colorado's underground workers, as various authorities noted in the late nineteenth century. One example illustrates that even minor injuries could have fatal consequences. The husband of Margie S. Alley was injured by falling rock in Ibex Mine on June 4, 1899. Alley was a subscriber to the Catholic hospital to which he was taken in an "express wagon." While in the hospital he contracted smallpox and subsequently died in the Leadville "pest house" on June 26. Miner Alley's experiences illustrate that secondary infection continued to be a problem for underground workers who were more likely to be seriously injured.[15]

Silicosis, mining's most insidious occupational disease, emerged in Colorado and elsewhere as working miners spent their lives underground. Medical and labor historian Alan Derickson defined silicosis as "a chronic respiratory disease that results from the inhalation of free silica (SiO_2) one of the primary constituents of the earth's crust. . . . Inhaling microscopic silica particles (of less than ten microns in diameter) for many years led to fibrotic scarring of the lungs. Fibrosis, in turn, led to impaired respiratory function and a predisposition to pulmonary tuberculosis and pneumonia." The disease posed special problems because the U.S. mining industry consistently rejected responsibility for the disease, and its respiratory manifestations were compounded in the high altitude of Colorado's mining camps.

The result was that miners with silicosis, or "miner's con," attempted to keep the symptoms secret lest a stigma attach to them. Mabel Barbee Lee vividly remembered her father's fits of coughing and gasping. The description she presents in *Cripple Creek Days* is still one of the most graphic: "He leaned far over, clutching his throat and choking for breath. It seemed as though he would never stop. His face turned purplish red and beads of perspiration stood out on his forehead." Although the careful analysis of the disease that led to its categorization as an occupational disease would await medical research in the twentieth century, Colorado miners exhibited the classic symptoms before the turn of the century. Given the medical knowledge of the time, victims of silicosis would likely have been treated as were patients with pneumonia or tuberculosis. This treatment would have proven ineffective, since medical research has identified silicosis as a progressive debilitation. Only actions taken to limit the creation of the dust or efforts to limit the intake of the particles could reduce the risk of miner's con.[16]

Colorado physicians began treating occupational injuries and diseases shortly before the extraordinary expansion of knowledge that occurred in the late nineteenth and early twentieth centuries. Colorado physicians benefited from experiences of the Civil War doctors who faced traumatic injuries on an unprecedented scale. Before the expansion of underground operations in the last quarter of the nineteenth century, Colorado doctors had effective anaesthesia and would learn about the importance of antiseptics in reducing or preventing secondary infections. The physicians faced a steady progression of injuries and illness, but the similarity of the conditions permitted doctors to improve effective intervention and to reexamine periodically less effective treatments. Silicosis alone defied their best efforts; certainly the other pulmonary-respiratory illnesses proved equally obstinate in this period. Even before the end of the century, miners began to associate the disease with the dust they breathed and the new technologies that magnified its effects. The new compressed air drills were referred to as "widow makers." Physicians may have suspected the connections, but they encountered more serious injuries and probably devoted more of their attention to ameliorating or remedying the suffering they believed it was within their power to affect.

Notes

1. U.S. Surgeon-General's Office, *The Medical and Surgical History of the War of the Rebellion (1861–1865). Prepared in Accordance With the Acts of Congress, Under the Direction of Surgeon General Joseph K. Barnes, United States Army* (Washington, D.C.: Government Printing Office, 1875–1883), 9 vols. See also George W. Adams, *Doctors in Blue* (New York: Henry Schuman, 1952); Stewart Brooks, *Civil War Medicine* (Springfield, Ill.: Charles C. Thomas,

1966); Horace H. Cunningham, *Doctors in Gray* (Baton Rouge: Louisiana State University Press, 1959); and Phyllis A. Stone, "The Patients' View of Civil War Medicine," M.A. Thesis, Southwest Texas State University, 1982.

2. Brooks, *Civil War Medicine*, 24–26; *The Statistical History of the United States From Colonial Times to the Present* (Stamford, Conn.: Fairfield, 1965), 34; Elizabeth Van Steenwyk, *Frontier Fever: The Silly, Superstitious—and Sometimes Sensible—Medicine of the Pioneers* (New York: Walker, 1995), 102–108.

3. Brooks, *Civil War Medicine*, 65–70.

4. Ronald C. Brown, *Hard-Rock Miners: The Intermountain West, 1860–1920* (College Station: Texas A&M University Press, 1979), Appendix B, 173–176; Diary of I. J. Baldwin, 1873–1874, Record of trip from Providence to San Francisco and return, typescript, 17, State Historical Society of Colorado, Denver. Bessie Launder Richards of St. Elmo, Colorado, remembered that her community had no resident physicians, and so the sick and injured nursed themselves or went to Buena Vista; Richards, "Mining Town Memories—Colorado and Mexico," typescript of interview conducted by Mel Erskine, Berkeley, 1967, Bancroft Library, University of California, Berkeley.

5. Brooks, *Civil War Medicine*, 77–88, 99–102; Van Steenwyk, *Frontier Fever*, 91–101, 106–108.

6. Diary of John A. Hitching, 60, Hitching Collection, Western History Collections, University of Colorado Libraries, Boulder, Colorado; Ray Colwell, "Cripple Creek: Some Recollections of My Boyhood There," manuscript, 10, in Alfred B. Colwell Collection, American Heritage Center, University of Wyoming, Laramie; Bureau of the Census and Social Science Research Council, *The Statistical History of the United States from Colonial Times to the Present* (Stamford, Conn.: Fairfield Publishers, Inc., 1965), Series D 785–792, 100.

7. Robert Livermore, "Twenty-Seven Years of Work and Fun in Mining," 8, paper presented to the Boston Section of the American Institute of Mining Engineers, 1935, in the Robert Livermore Papers, American Heritage Center, University of Wyoming, Laramie.

8. Kenneth L. Fahnestock to Thomas F. Daly, Leadville, June 6, 1899, Letterbook 7, 482, in John F. Campion Papers, Western History Collection, University of Colorado, Boulder; A. C. (Arthur Cecil) Todd, *The Cornish Miner in America: The Contribution to the Mining History of the United States by Emigrant Cornish Miners—The Men Called Cousin Jacks* (Glendale, Calif.: Clark, 1967), 164–165.

9. Alfred Castner King, *Mountain Idylls and Other Poems* (New York: F. H. Revell, 1901), 9–10, 48–49; "Minutes of the Creede Pioneer Society of Denver, 1918–1958," 56, in State Historical Society of Colorado, Denver.

10. "Notice of Accident Made by Chas. Bargler," November 13, 1901, Letterbook 8, 266, in Campion Papers; "Diary" of Cecil C. Morgan, February 5, 1878, in Western History Department, Denver Public Library; "Robert Livermore: An Autobiography," typescript, 80, in Robert Livermore Papers, American Heritage Center, University of Wyoming, Laramie (n.d.).

11. Livermore, "Work and Fun in Mining," 8–9; Kenneth L. Fahnestock to Thomas

F. Daly, Leadville, August 13, 1902, Letterbook 8, in Campion Papers.

12. S. W. Mudd to H. A. Lee, Commissioner of Mines, May 9, 1900, Leadville, Letterbook 7, and "Ibex Accident Report to the Commissioner of Miners," prepared by Kenneth L. Fahnestock, October 31, 1900, Leadville, Letterbook 8, in Campion Papers.

13. Anna Feageans to John F. Campion, September 8, 1905, Chicago, in Correspondence 1905, and Campion to Feageans, September 15, 1905, Denver, in Letterbook (1904–1906), 139; Report of P.B., December 29, 1900, Detective Reports; and Copy, Kenneth L. Fahnestock to Thomas F. Daly, May 5, 1903, and August 17, 1903, Leadville, Letterbook 8, 461, and 487, in Campion Papers.

14. Dairy of Elizabeth D. Sayre, December 15 and 16, 1889, in Hal Sayre Papers, Western History Collection, University of Colorado, Boulder; Copies, Kenneth L. Fahnestock to Thomas F. Daly, Leadville, July 14 and 28, 1898, in Letterbook 7, 143, and 170, and July 6, 1907, in Letterbook 8, 692; Copy, Fahnestock to George F. Campion, Leadville, March 22, 1905, in Letterbook 3 of Fahnestock, 231; Report of Death of James A. Sullivan, September 7, 1898, in Letterbook 7, 218, in Campion Papers; Frank A. Crampton, *Deep Enough: A Working Stiff in the Western Mine Camps* (Denver: Sage Books, 1956), 42–43.

15. Fahnestock to Daly, May 26 and December 5, 1899, and John F. Campion to Mrs. Margie S. Alley, September 26, 1899, in Letterbook 7, 264, 717, and 653, in Campion Papers.

16. Alan Derickson, *Workers' Health, Workers' Democracy: The Western Miners' Struggle, 1891–1925* (Ithaca: Cornell University Press, 1988), 39–52, quote on 39; Brown, *Hard-Rock Miners*, 93–94; Mabel Barbee Lee, *Cripple Creek Days* (New York: Doubleday, 1958), 63, 68–70, 184, 220–222, quote on 68.

Photographic Essay

O VER 2,000 YEARS AGO Greek physician Hippocrates wrote: "Medicine is the most distinguished of all the arts, but through the ignorance of those who practice it, and of those who casually judge such practitioners, it is now of all the arts by far the least esteemed." The "father of medicine" could just as easily have been describing medicine in the mining West 150 years ago or 80 years ago.

Many physicians who practiced in the mining camps had subscribed to Hippocrates's oath; some had likely never heard of it. Their patients could only hope for the best: "I will use treatment to help the sick according to my ability and judgment."

Photographs of the medical profession are nearly as rare as a bonanza discovery. Views of hospitals appear fairly regularly; they boosted civic pride and give the viewer a sense of community development—something all local boosters wanted. Beyond that medical photos are difficult to find, except for those of individual physicians.

The photographs that follow take you back to a medical time that cannot be called modern. Photography and cameras matured more than medicine did during the years under examination. Study these photos as you would any other primary source with an understanding, yet critical eye; they have much to tell us beyond the first quick visual image.

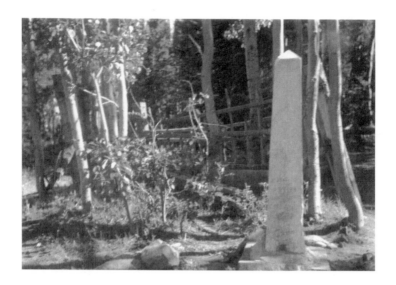

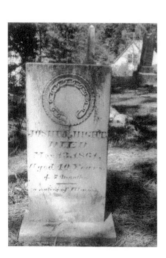

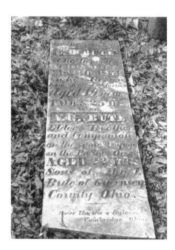

In hundreds of long forgotten western cemeteries and even more unmarked graves lie the remains of miners and their families. They mark the course of the empire and the westward march of disease and death. Much can be learned about the medical history of the West by reading the inscriptions on tombstones. They recount the story but not the tragedy and sadness.

Samuel and Margaret Richards of Caribou, Colorado, lost three children—Anna, Willie, and Margaret, July 5, 6, and 8, 1879—during a diphtheria epidemic.

The Bute brothers died coming home from California, one at sea and the other of yellow fever at Grand Gulf, Mississippi, only a few hundred miles from their Ohio home.

Joshua Hight died far from his native Illinois in Allegany, California. At age forty his dream ended, as it did for so many others, far short of the fortune he hoped to find.

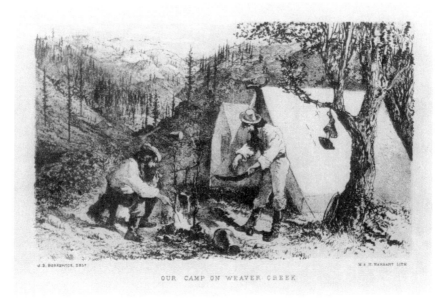

OUR CAMP ON WEAVER CREEK

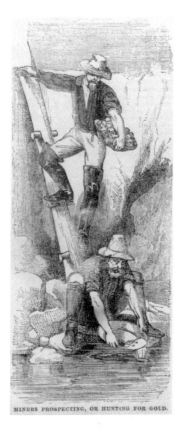

MINERS PROSPECTING, OR HUNTING FOR GOLD.

Early prospectors and miners often camped near their claims (*above*). This practice could be conducive to good health or could break the individual's health; both happened in the mining West. Courtesy J. D. Borthwick, *Three Years in California* (1857).

California miners at work (*left*); the accompanying story observed about placer mining: "It is no boys' play: . . . unless a man possess an iron constitution, he is almost sure to give way under its hardships. The fever and ague he is almost sure to encounter, and this will 'shake' the flesh off his limbs and sides with most miraculous speed." Courtesy *Gleason's Pictorial . . . Companion* (1852).

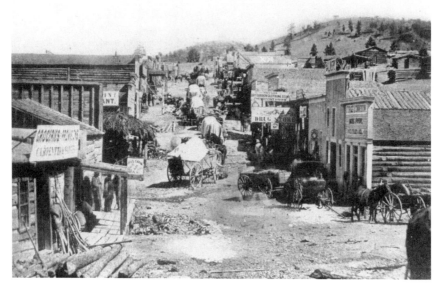

Hastily built, littered with trash, often unsanitary, and crowded, mining camps and towns awaited the fortune seekers; Helena, Montana, 1865. Courtesy Montana Historical Society.

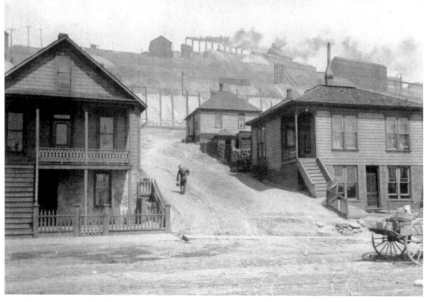

Smelter towns added a variety of smoke and respiratory problems to the local environment; one of the worst was Butte, Montana, in the 1890s. Courtesy Special Collections, Colorado College.

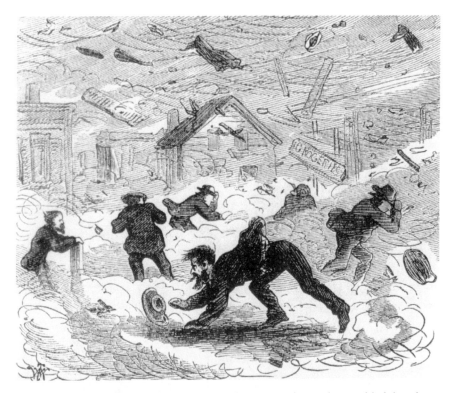

The mining West provided a climatic kaleidoscope to those who gambled their lives to find their bonanza; the Washoe Zephyr was famous in Virginia City, Nevada. Courtesy Mark Twain, *Roughing It* (1872).

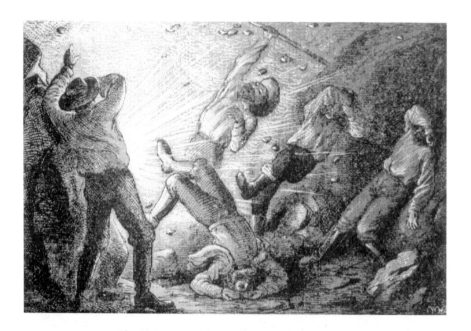

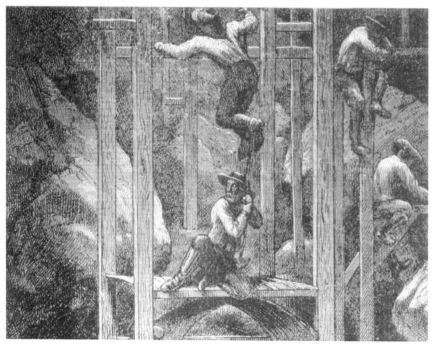

Every time a miner goes underground he faces danger and death; these drawings of Comstock accidents illustrate the hazards. Courtesy Dan DeQuille, *The Big Bonanza* (1876).

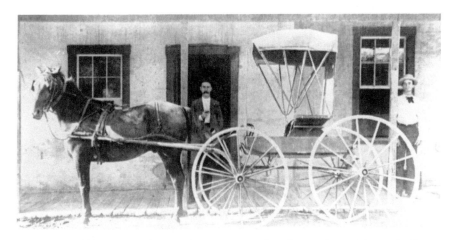

"Who shall decide when doctors disagree?" wondered writer/poet Alexander Pope. For mining camp doctors like John C. Handy, that was seldom a worry—he was the only doctor available. Courtesy Arizona Historical Foundation, Arizona State University, Tempe, Arizona.

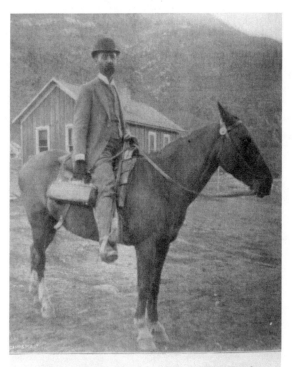

C. F. & I. Surgeon at Redstone Making His Daily Rounds.

Company doctors served many mines and camps— Colorado Fuel and Iron Dr. A. Taylor at Redstone, Colorado, carries the ever-present black bag. Courtesy Denver Public Library, Western History Department.

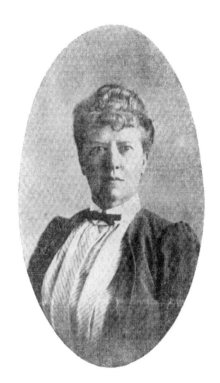

California and Nevada physician and famous Goldfield pioneer and mine owner Frances E. Williams. Courtesy Nevada Historical Society.

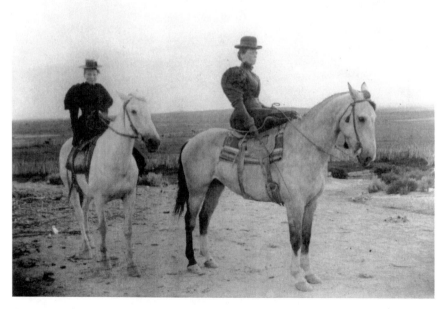

Some mining camps had only a midwife to help women with the birth of their children; Hilda Erickson (front) was one of those in Utah. Used by permission, Utah State Historical Society, all rights reserved.

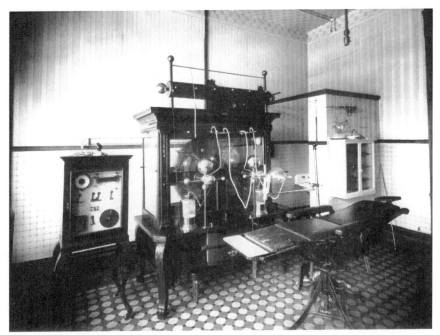

Dr. George Harding's office in Salt Lake City awaits a patient; this is larger and more spacious than many doctors' offices.

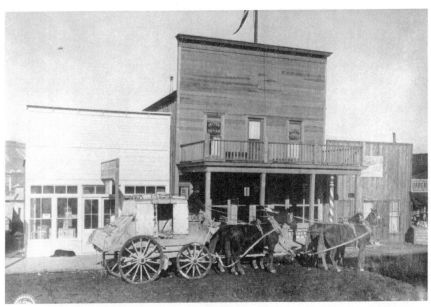

The Goldfield stage stopped next to the offices of Doctors Turner and Rhyan; this false-front building is typical of mining community architecture. Courtesy Nevada Historical Society.

Many miners and mining camp residents relied on almanacs such as this one or on patent medicines as their first line of medical treatment. Courtesy Duane A. Smith.

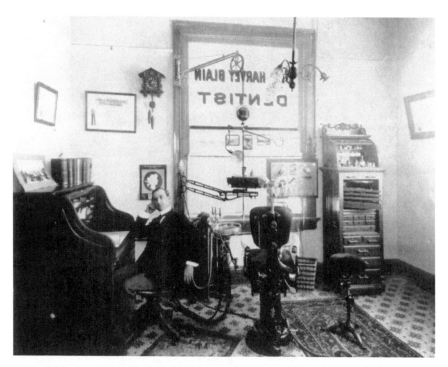

Dr. Harvey Blain of Prescott, Arizona, pauses "thoughtfully" at 1:15 in the afternoon while awaiting a customer; he used a pump drill to work on patients' teeth. Courtesy Arizona Historical Foundation, Arizona State University, Tempe, Arizona.

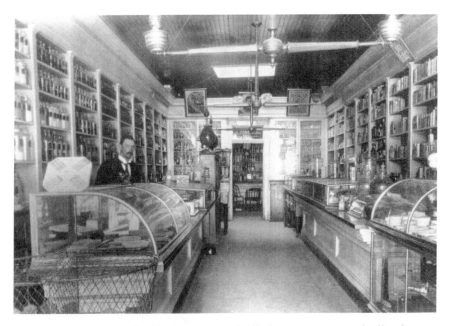

A Virginia City, Nevada, drugstore in 1898 filled prescriptions and offered many "over-the-counter" medicines to attempt to aid sufferers with real or imaginary ills. Courtesy Nevada Historical Society.

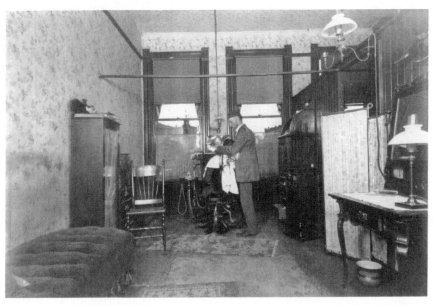

Most Americans were unfamiliar with the toothbrush, and their mouths were dental disasters waiting to happen; Dr. Richardson of Helena, Montana, treats a patient. Courtesy Denver Public Library, Western History Department.

Hospitals not only served a medical need; they displayed how far towns had developed and matured like their eastern cousins. Many larger mining towns had hospitals; extremely few of the smaller mining camps were so fortunate.

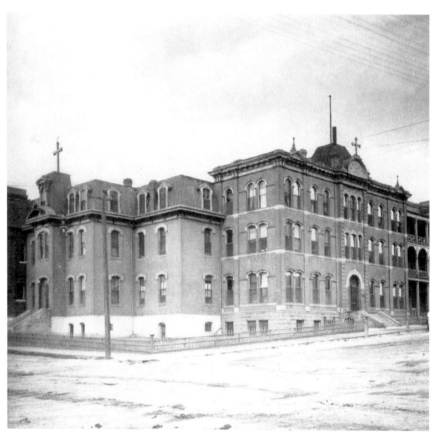

St. James Hospital, Butte, Montana, one of the state's best. Courtesy Montana Historical Society.

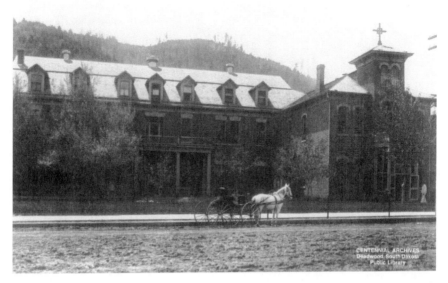

St. Joseph's Hospital, Deadwood, South Dakota, opened in 1878. Courtesy Deadwood Public Library.

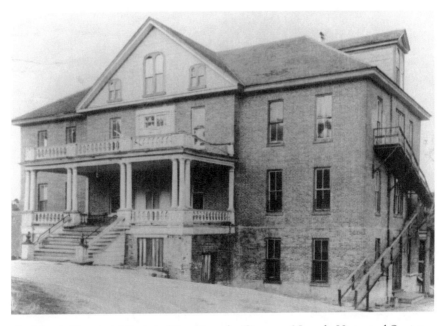

St. Mary's Hospital, Virginia City, Nevada. Courtesy Nevada Historical Society.

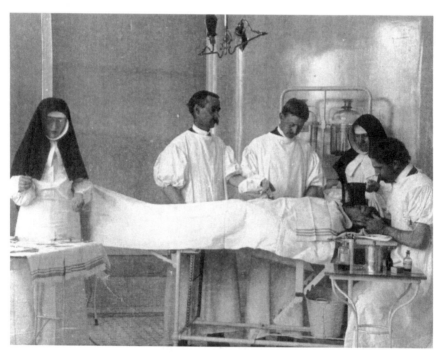

The Sisters of St. Francis prepare a patient for an operation; they worked as nurses in this Colorado Springs hospital, as did other Catholic orders throughout the mining West. Courtesy Colorado Historical Society.

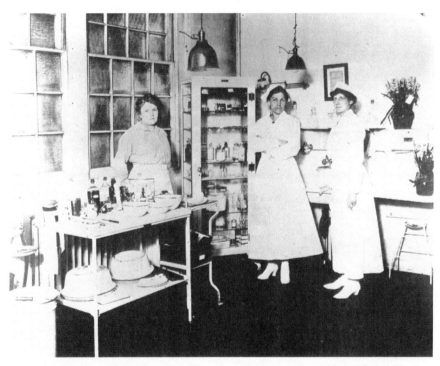

The Ouray, Colorado, hospital, built by the city, was later operated by the Sisters of Mercy and finally became a private hospital. This appears a formidable trio of nurses; but as "Mr. Dooley" said about doctors and medicine, "It wudden't make anny diff'rence which ye called in—if ye had a good nurse." Courtesy Ouray Historical Society.

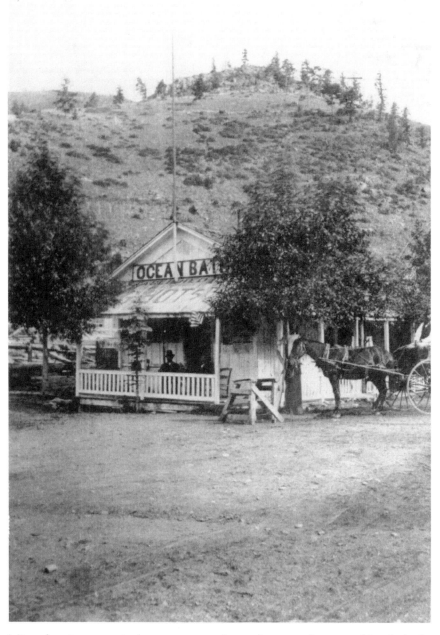

Mineral springs promised a menagerie of miracle cures if one would only bath, drink, or rest awhile; some mining districts, such as Idaho Springs, Colorado, had them next door. Courtesy Special Collections, Colorado College.

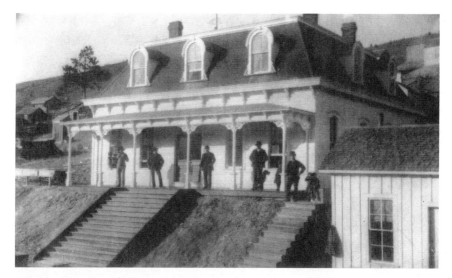

The Homestake Company provided medical benefits for its workers as early as 1878; this hospital was built in 1886. Courtesy Homestake Mining Company.

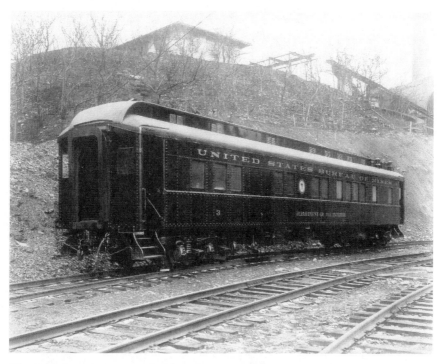

The U.S. Bureau of Mines developed special railroad "safety cars" to provide safety training for miners and to render technical support and trained personnel during mining disasters. Bureau of Mines Safety Car #3, courtesy National Archives.

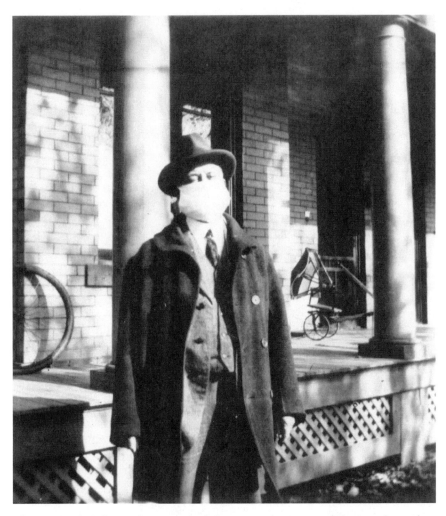

The 1918–1919 flu epidemic proved the worst the mining West confronted; it seemed especially deadly for people living at higher elevations. How much good these masks accomplished can be questioned. Courtesy Montana Historical Society.

6

"Wearing Out, Not Rusting Out"

REST OF THE WEST

CALIFORNIA, NEVADA, AND COLORADO incited a mining frenzy that spread throughout nearly the entire West. Prospectors and miners invaded Idaho and Montana in the early 1860s, then moved into Utah in the face of Mormon opposition. The Spanish had opened mines in Arizona and New Mexico a century earlier, but when Americans reached the region, the industry gained a new intensity. The Black Hills of South Dakota lured the adventuresome in the 1870s, and the more unlikely Wyoming and eastern Oregon also briefly held some promise of golden wealth.

The medical problems these immigrants encountered were not unfamiliar. Potatoes hauled in on men's backs curbed a scurvy outbreak in the winter of 1861–1862 in Oro Fino, Idaho. James Knox Polk Miller recorded incidents of exposure, headaches, homesickness (more common than would have been expected), aches and pains, and overindulgence in "spirits" during his 1865–1867 stay in Virginia City, Montana. Wickenburg, Arizona, residents suffered through a fever and chills epidemic in 1867. Neuralgia, alcohol, accidents, colds, and wintry weather plagued the 1868 miners in South Pass City and Miner's Delight, Wyoming.

Smallpox visited Deadwood, South Dakota, in the summer of 1876, and diphtheria plagued residents a few years later. Prospector/miner Richard Hughes's diary registered only a cut thumb and hard work to mark his first ten months in the Black Hills, whereas Estelline Bennett recalled pneumonia and mountain fever in her youth. Silver City, New Mexico, endured a smallpox scare in 1877; residents raised money to vaccinate youngsters and adults who did not have "this safeguard." In 1879–1880 the children of Silver Reef, Utah, came down with scarlet fever and whooping cough in larger than usual numbers. Of a different nature, sunstroke and heat exhaustion claimed more victims in Arizona mining communities than anywhere else. Park City, Utah, confronted a diphtheria outbreak in the fall of 1880; residents were pleased when it did not recur the next year.

Contaminated water caused dysentery and diarrhea among Tombstone, Arizona, residents.[1]

As elsewhere in the mining West, lack of sanitation created much of the trouble. Newspapers and some residents worked to improve conditions, with varying results. In May 1866 the editor of the *Owyhee Avalanche* (Ruby City, Idaho) chastised merchants and individuals for letting "offal and other filth" accumulate in their neighborhoods. Editors in Deadwood in 1877, in Pinal, Arizona, four years later, and in Butte, Montana, in 1883 pleaded for a healthier environment. When myriad complaints about Park City's "deplorable" sanitary conditions and the most "disgusting stenches imaginable" failed to bring improvements, the *Park Record* (June 5, 1880) warned, "If people will continue to breed disease, they must not complain if diphtheria or other illnesses carries off their little ones."

In all these trials and tribulations, very little could be called new and strange, although previous experience did not guarantee preventive action. Americans in these places and times too often were careless with local sanitation until an epidemic shocked them to their senses. The prevailing attitude that these mining communities were only temporary homes further undermined concern, whether in California in the 1840s or in New Mexico in the 1880s. Physicians had little success in overcoming reluctance to spend the time and money needed to solve a communitywide problem. Both children and adults paid a heavy price for that indifference.

As the years went by, however, more interest arose in establishing hospitals, especially in the larger mining towns. A familiar pattern began to unfold. The county built one hospital for Deadwood, and a Catholic Sisters order founded a hospital in Silver Reef. Women in Globe, Arizona, conducted a subscription drive to purchase a building and provide furnishings. Doctors occasionally opened their own facilities, and miners' unions sometimes answered the call if no other group jumped in to supply the need. There is no way of judging whether these institutions provided care equal to that found elsewhere. Here, too, the sick and injured seemed reluctant to avail themselves of the services. Hospitals had not yet escaped their nineteenth-century stigmas.

"Awakened in the night by a raging tooth ache and suffered till time to call a dentist," noted Tombstone's George Parsons. He persisted through two dentists before a third successfully removed an ulcerated wisdom tooth. As did most mining camp residents throughout the West, he waited until pain drove him to seek professional help. Luckily for Parsons, Tombstone provided resident dentists; so did most of the mining towns, like Silver City, Idaho, and Butte. Mining camps generally did not.

The traveling dentist remained a popular expedient in the camps and even in some towns. Dentist R. F. Burgess of Los Angeles stopped at Globe's

Central Hotel and told readers of the *Silver Belt* (October 25, 1879) that he was "prepared to do all kinds of work." Park City advertised for a "good dentist, who thoroughly understands his business." The newspaper hoped he would be "conscientious enough not to charge fancy prices just because this is a mining town."[2]

High medical and dental costs, urban congestion, and an alluring environment where accidents waited around every corner assured that parents faced considerable challenges in raising their children to adulthood. In a time when each family was, by tradition, expected to have four children—one for each parent, one for natural increase of the population, and one who would die—illness and death abided as constant companions.

Children were pioneers, too, in populating the West. They came with the forty-niners and the fifty-niners. Chicagoan Dr. Charles Clark empathized with the children he saw in 1860 on his way to Pike's Peak country: "The little children were objects for pity, harmless and helpless as they were, confined to the limits of the wagon night and day; sometimes parched by heat, sometimes shivering with cold, and often suffering from the want of water." He concluded that any father who would subject his family to such hardship earned "*non compos mentis*" status.

Louise Clapp looked around her Rich Bar, California, home and wrote her sister, "This is an awful place for children; and nervous mothers would 'die daily' if they could see little Mary running fearless to the very edge of, and looking down into, these holes—many of them sixty feet in depth." Nervous mothers probably did not remain long in a mining community environment!

Nearly all identifiable children's diseases descended on the mining towns and camps. Measles, scarlet fever, typhus, and smallpox were transmitted mainly through personal contact. Dysentery spread through contact with the ill, their clothes and personal items, and fouled water. Meningitis, or "brain fever," whooping cough, and intestinal diseases circulated at will in urban settings. Fevers took hold in a variety of ways and forms. The greatest child killer, diphtheria, was passed quickly through the air or by touch; it is estimated to have caused one childhood death in four. Diphtheria hit both the very young and those in their teens; no parent ever felt safe from this dreaded disease.

A child's life was most in jeopardy during its first five years, a circumstance typical for the rest of the nation as well. The lack of public sanitation (a breeding cesspool for childhood diseases), the often crowded living conditions, and squalid housing exacerbated parents' concerns. The fact that doctors were practicing in most of the mining towns, if not in all the mining camps, helped to counteract some of the worst conditions.

Mary Hallock Foote expressed the feeling of many mothers when she twice battled the fever that nearly cost her her young son, Boykin. During the first bout she watched over him day and night, "every two hours a tablespoonful of milk forced between the fever-crusted lips, every four hours the shuddering dose of raw quinine dissolved in water." The second time, aided by Leadville's Dr. Frederick D'Avignon, who prescribed "mercury and jalap," Boykin again recovered, but the struggle took a terrible toll on his mother: "My nerves were undone for the rest of the summer and my sleep destroyed by the panic-terrors of that illness."

Foote had been "rattled and convulsed with fear" because she had never nursed such a serious illness. Mothers and fathers, too, acquired that experience very quickly in the mining West.[3]

Doctors tried their best, but their lack of understanding of the causes of illness and the general state of the profession in the last decades of the century hampered them. Calomel and a variety of "aromatic powders" prescribed for dysentery proved of questionable value. To attempt to keep a diphtheria victim's throat open, physicians tried diluted sulfuric acid and other concoctions that used salt, pepper, vinegar, and other more exotic ingredients. Inhalation of the fumes of sulphur, turpentine, tar, and brimstone also had adherents as a favorite cure. Doctors occasionally attempted tracheotomies, a dangerous procedure under the operating conditions of the day.

Gargling with a solution of chlorate of potash or a little glycerine and spraying with a mixture of iodine or chloride of iron with glycerine were procedures recommended for sore throats. Quarantine sometimes helped to control the spread of diseases, but more often they rampaged with appalling speed. Bed rest, a warm bath at night, and a drop of ipecac syrup in water every hour or two supposedly comforted the influenza patient. By the 1890s cleanliness, warmth, and fresh air in the sick room, along with pure water and proper food for the patient, were being promoted by physicians and by such home medical books as *The New American Family Physician*. Without question, these ideas provided a major step in the right direction.

Although illnesses struck more fear in parents' hearts, accidents probably claimed more victims. The inviting mine tunnels, ponds, and shafts, nearby streams, and hills all beckoned young adventurers. Runaway wagons and horses, fireworks, construction sites, rough-and-tumble games, trash dumps, and abandoned buildings held both great allure and potential danger; so did the red-light district, although in a different way. The numerous relics and discards of the mining industry—such as ore cars, blasting caps, machinery, tools, and dumps—gave opportunity for adventure and accident. Limited only by their active imaginations, the young of the mining communities could find something dangerous everywhere around them on which to expend their considerable energy.

To the reader it might appear a miracle that any children survived to their teenage years, but many did. John Waldorf spoke for these stalwarts when he wrote about his childhood years on the Comstock: "To be raised in a mining camp means an experience as full of thrills and wounds and scars as going to the wars." An entire chapter is filled with his adventures, most of which would have turned parents' hair gray had they known about them. Deadwood's Estelline Bennett remembered her youth: "There never was but one Deadwood . . . flared highest and brightest." Mabel Barbee Lee would not have exchanged her life at Cripple Creek: "Cripple Creek to me was anything but a godforsaken hole. It opened out as a world of mysterious, fascinating adventure, waiting for me to explore its every hill, gulch and alley!" Nor would Morris Parker of White Oaks, New Mexico, have substituted another home for the one of his youth. He reminisced about the "good old days, days of trial and change, of give and take, when friendship was deep and sincere."

Dan De Quille emphatically refuted the notion that "children should not be reared there," referring to Virginia City. He judged that they "grow like mushrooms" and concluded that "finer or more robust children can be seen in no town or city in the Union." Although the adventuresome life was a child's delight, it was always tempered by the stress its dangers created for conscientious parents.[4]

Mothers undoubtedly worried more than fathers, who tended to be more involved in outside work than in child rearing at home. The women also had personal concerns. From their arrival, they encountered both old and new health problems. Unlike their rural sisters, however, they generally found nearby female companionship, midwives, and doctors. Nonetheless, a dismayed Californian, Mary Ballou, wrote that she would not advise women to come west and suffer the "toil and fatigue that I have suffered for the sake of a little gold; neither do I advise any one to come." A friend gloomily lamented, "Oh dear I am so homesick that I must die." But they came anyway, rather than suffer separation from loved ones, and stayed to make a home.

One of women's major concerns in the West, as it had been in the East, was finding themselves in a "family way." Even under the best of nineteenth-century conditions, this aspect of the "female ritual" could be life threatening. An estimated one of every thirty mothers died giving birth; others suffered from depression and anxiety. Pregnancy and birth called for the support of other women, something the mining communities could provide. Neighboring women aided each other in many ways, from providing physical care to minding children and discussing birth control methods.

Doctors and midwives commonly tended the mother through childbirth, but if neither was available delivery could become a family matter. If inexperienced or unskilled, the attenders could cause injury to the baby or the mother. Women endured vaginal tears, prolapsed uteruses, and painful hernias, along with sore breasts and milk fever. The babies suffered a variety of traumas, from brain damage to infections. A stillborn child created great emotional and physical distress and was not an uncommon occurrence (accounting for roughly 5 percent of births).

Grief over the death of a baby was difficult to express in letters. Susanna Townsend attempted it when she wrote to her sisters about the death of her month-old daughter, Ellen Beulah:

> If I were near you I could tell you so many of her little winning ways, and how very pretty and cunning she was.
>
>   These are little things to write perhaps you think who have had so many babies, but I think we must be excused if we were a little extra delighted with our baby being you know rather *old folks* [mid-thirties] to have the first one. At any rate we did feel very happy with her all the time she was with us and it was hard to part with her.

A stillborn baby followed, but Susanna eventually bore three daughters who lived.

Mining community mothers did not have the luxury of a long recuperation after childbirth; in the eastern United States a month or more was typical. Unless she was extremely ill or wealthy enough to afford help, the mother resumed her domestic duties in a much shorter period—perhaps within a few days—and took on the additional role of nurse/physician, as already discussed.[5]

In late Victorian America birth control, along with sex, remained a taboo subject for general discussion. The so-called Comstock laws (named after Anthony Comstock) made it illegal to mail contraceptive or sex information, thereby driving this aspect of women's culture underground. More female physicians could have helped with this problem because many women remained reluctant to discuss these delicate issues with men, even doctors. As a result, mothers, older women, and friends dealt with the topic. Mary Hallock Foote wrote her friend Helena Gilder in December 1876 about a "sure way of limiting one's family." She had received the news from her sister-in-law, Mary Hague:

> It sounds perfectly revolting, but one must face anything rather than the inevitable result of Nature's methods. At all events there is nothing injurious about this. Mrs. Hague is a very fastidious woman and I hardly think she would submit to anything very bad. These things are called "cundums" and are made either of rubber or skin.

They could be purchased, Foote went on to say, from all first-class druggists.

The burden of birth control fell to the women. Beyond the late-appearing condoms, they could also use diaphragms, douches, and one book's recommendation of a "delicate piece of sponge moistened with water" that "immediately afterwards was to be withdrawn by a very narrow ribbon attached to it." The only objection the author could see was that "the woman had to leave the bed [for] a few moments." Withdrawal, the rhythm method, and abstinence also had practitioners, as did some folk ideas, including the use of petroleum jelly ("a greased egg won't hatch") and the idea (hope!) that nursing a baby prevented ovulation and thus pregnancy.

No method was foolproof, and individual decisions about which to use had to be weighed carefully. The medical profession could dispense help and advice about birth control, as could a midwife or neighbor, but ultimately the decision rested with the individuals directly involved.

That paladin of virtue Anthony Comstock, the leading "pornography" fighter of the generation, and his supporters attempted to suppress discussion of birth control, without success. Home medical books began to treat the subject more openly. In 1864 Alvin Chase had recommended that married women write to him about "subjects not introduced" in his book. A generation later, *The New American Family Physician* included an entire section on "pregnancy and confinement." Menopause was often welcomed as the end to childbearing years; as one woman noted, "one thing that was nice, after you went through menopause, you didn't have to worry."[6]

Abortion was an option also available to women. Until the 1870s abortion remained a legal, although medically hazardous, procedure, and the number of aborted pregnancies may have been as high as 20 percent of all pregnancies. Abortifacients such as "ergot, oil of tansy, and black hellebore" were used, as were the services of abortionists. A coalition of medical doctors, religious authorities, and moral reformers curbed this means of terminating unwanted pregnancies through legislation.

From that decade abortion was transformed from an acceptable practice into a "sin." Dr. T. J. Ritter, in discouraging its use, wrote, "I say nothing of the sin. I leave that to those who ought to teach these things to the young while they are yet in the formative period of life." Despite his pleas and those of others, abortion continued, "notorious and extremely prevalent," as late as the turn of the twentieth century. Women from all classes of society, married and unmarried, could search out an abortionist once they had made the right contacts. The prevalence of abortion in the mining communities is unknown. That subject was buried deep among the topics about which genteel Victorians did not write or talk publicly.

As discussed earlier, the shortage of women physicians produced a distinct void that deterred women from discussing their problems with a doctor. Occasionally, however, a male doctor could be found who specialized in women's illnesses. Remember, Dr. A. B. Spinney, for instance, advertised that he was impressed with "the delicacy of the subject" and could assure his "lady patients" of "immediate relief." The catalog of ills he successfully treated included "nervousness, neuralgia, loss of appetite, vaginal irregularities, indigestion and many petty irritating distractions." Consultations cost nothing.[7]

Another class of women in the mining communities found themselves even farther removed from medical attention—the prostitutes. They obviously did not practice abstinence and interruption as methods of birth control. Women of ill repute sought out abortionists much more often than did their married sisters from respectable homes. The girls of the line knew well the various means to abort and did so with alacrity when the need arose. The "fair but frail" also encountered another plague of their profession their "good" sisters hoped to avoid—social diseases.

"Thirty seconds of Venus, a lifetime of mercury," was one Victorian admonition. Syphilis and gonorrhea may have been more prevalent than contemporary sources were willing to admit. Mining town newspapers undeniably carried ads for patent medicine "cures" and for doctors who promised a "cure." The volume of advertising said more about the problem than any direct commentary.

Self-described as "celebrated for [having achieved] thousands of cures," Dr. Young of San Francisco promised his patients a "cure guaranteed or no pay." Mild cases could be relieved in "two to five days"; others took somewhat longer, including "old, chronic, mercurial, syphilitic and all private diseases." Some communities promoted their own "specialists." At Pioche, Dr. D. H. Whepley "guaranteed a sure cure in cases of venereal disease." Chinese doctors were famous throughout the West for healing such maladies. The commonly used mercury produced its own side effects and, like other remedies, treated only the symptoms, not the cause.

No cure was available to this generation, no doubt explaining the reason for such strong opposition to the red-light districts. As one author bluntly stated, "Syphilis affects most public and clandestine or secret prostitutes. It can best be prevented by avoiding all chance of infection." Social diseases constituted a veiled corner of Victorian morals and medicine. Many innocent people could suffer when an infected man "[sowed] his wild oats."

Another "curse" of the red-light district was drug addiction. Although medical men understood addiction's potential dangers by the 1880s, not until the 1890s did it become a matter of general concern. Painkillers, patent medicines, cocaine-enhanced palliatives (marvelously adapted to the tonic trade), morphine, and opium held the potential for addiction. They were prescribed and purchased freely over the druggist's counter, drunk in popular beverages (Celery Kola and Coca-Cola), and used to lace patent medicines, including children's cough syrup.

Addicts, whose addictions stemmed from both medical and nonmedical causes, surfaced in all walks of life. In the nineteenth century the former clearly constituted the majority, in part because some doctors used morphine to end alcoholic addiction, believing it the lesser of two evils. Then, in the 1860s and 1870s hypodermic medication came into fashion, giving physicians a powerful and faster way to provide opiate relief.

Opium smoking constituted the most prevalent form of nonmedical addiction and remained confined almost exclusively to the far West until the 1870s. It came with Chinese laborers, eventually spread to the white underworld, and from there moved eastward. Smoking in a "den" or "dive" or at home held an important attraction other methods of opiate use lacked: the opportunity for social interaction. Alfred Doten casually mentioned in his diary that he visited Mary, who seems to have been a prostitute, and smoked opium with her. It was a way to relax and join with friends in a congenial atmosphere. Opium dens most visibly manifested this type of nonmedical use in the mining communities. The Chinese became the targets of much abuse, but non-Chinese patronized these drug havens as well.

Such activities illustrated this insidious and often secret segment of American life. An occasional article mentioned a "drug fiend," and the press sometimes featured an "outrage" story.

Americans, ever the entrepreneurs, seized on ways to profit from the rehabilitation of victims of drug use and social diseases. Physicians concocted cures, and patent remedies proliferated. "Syphilene the magic remedy" promised a syphilis cure in twenty to sixty days, and Denver doctors Betts and Betts assured a "certain and positive cure for the awful effects of early vice." "The world [could] be thankful" that sixty Keeley Institutes opened in the United States, including several in the mining regions. Their "Double Chloride of Gold Remedies" ensured a miracle to "cure the liquor, opium, morphine, and tobacco habits." The founders warned readers about "fraudulent" establishments using similar titles.[8]

The Keeley approach gave ample evidence of the variety of addictions and the attention they were receiving. American medicine was slowly progressing by 1900, but that progress came too late to help the early addicts. The "cold turkey" withdrawal method of treatment, augmented by supportive therapy and/or sedation, for example, customarily promised a "cure" in two to four weeks. Astonishingly, the treatments often relied on opium, morphine, or codeine to effect cures. A study of the twenty most widely advertised cures found all but one included morphine. That one, the double chloride of gold the Keeley Institute used, contained no gold at all! Gold, combined with arsenic, iodine, bromine, or mercury, happened to be in vogue at the time as a cure for addiction.

These remedies rarely produced the promised results. This generation, however, was the first to wrestle with this problem, and it took more years of experience before the nature of this addiction was understood. In fact, the problem has still not been conquered.

Drugs also emerged as a vehicle for suicide (poisons had a following, too), serving as a particularly painless way of putting the sadness, bleakness, and misery of the red-light district behind. Nettie Moore in Virginia City, Montana, and Deadwood's Katie Smith and Mabel (last name unknown) all took that way out. Doctors with stomach pumps and antidotes rushed to save the intended victims; their success depended on the dosage ingested and their time of arrival.

Physicians were also called upon to correct the mistakes of druggists. Through ignorance or carelessness, druggists could easily err in filling out prescriptions. One letter writer labeled them "quack druggists" and called for a state examination. Drugstores displayed a variety of drugs for sale, including narcotics, stimulants, and sedatives, for as little as a nickel for a few grains. Unlabeled bottles in home medicine chests could be another source of potential danger. Dr. Chase cautioned his readers to insist that the druggist "in all cases" label medicine: "In this way you will not only save *money*, but perhaps *life*." Arsenic, laudanum, and similar items should "always be put where children cannot get at them." This was sound advice then as now.[9]

Areas blessed with salubrious climates boasted of their contributions to improved health. Arizona and New Mexico soon promoted themselves as beneficial relocation sites for people suffering from everything from catarrh to consumption. Colorado and California had already entered the competition for attracting consumptives and others, and Nevada and Montana lagged just a step behind. The combination of pure air, ozone, dryness, and invigorating climate would surely cure the "lungers." The simple promise of a prolonged life and the possible eradication of afflictions caught the attention of consumptives and sufferers of other respiratory ailments, who thronged to these new meccas. One ecstatic visitor wrote:

> [The climate] so far as pertains to health and longevity, seems at present to enlist the attention of nearly every one. It has come to be idolized by some as the land where time never wipes the roses from the cheeks of youth; the land where none grow old . . . the land where the fell destroyer, disease, has never stricken robust manhood, laid its blight upon effeminate womanhood, nor withered the hopes of frail childhood; but where the invalid in quest of health is reinvigorated and restored.

This wonderful environment combined with a hot springs multiplied the anticipated benefits. The "Celebrated Hot Springs of Southern New Mexico," for example, proffered all the atmospheric blessings and the "medicinal power of the waters." Nervousness, dizziness, coughs, chronic diseases, and debility "are speedily cured." Mining communities sought to join in the health stampede, but their isolation, industrial pollution, and high altitude deterred the ill. The more accessible and larger towns, like Tucson and Denver, generally grabbed the bulk of the business. As a health mecca, however, the region prospered.[10]

The failure of the mining camps and towns to attract the "one-lunged army" could be attributed to their unhealthful reputations. Butte stands out as a classic example of contaminated air, perhaps the region's worst. In the 1890s it became symbolic of industrial pollution.

Butte, in the last quarter of the nineteenth century, evolved from a gold to a silver and then a copper district. In the last stage it became world famous, as well as infamous. By 1889 Butte had acquired six "of the most modern and potent" smelters in the world along the base of its hill of copper and a population of 10,000. "The thicker the fumes the greater our financial vitality, and Butteites feel best when the fumes are thickest," bragged the *Butte Miner*. To make matters worse, heap roasting in the open air belched smoke from smoldering piles of copper ore.

These sulphur, arsenic, and copper fumes killed grass, flowers, and trees; cats that licked the grime off their fur risked arsenic poisoning. Some people argued that the smoke produced not only a financial blessing but also a healthful miracle. Mining engineer James Hague received a letter from F. E. Sargeant, who said "La Grippe" was raging in Butte, although in a much milder form than elsewhere: "It is the opinion of physicians that the sulphur smoke which permeates everywhere has a discouraging effect upon the microbe and causes it to relax its grip." William Andrews Clark, who became a millionaire thanks to Butte copper, made even more outrageous claims: "I say it would be a great deal better for other cities in the territory [Montana] if they had more smoke and less diphtheria and other diseases. It has been believed by all the physicians of Butte that the smoke which sometimes prevails there is a disinfectant, and destroys the microbes that constitute the germs of disease."

The reality was more grim. Smoke enveloped the community and the daily lives of its residents. From July through October 1890, 192 deaths were recorded, most from pneumonia and typhoid. In December 36 deaths were attributed to respiratory diseases. These deaths made a hollow mockery of the claims for the healthful qualities of smelter smoke.[11]

Finally facing the facts, Butte took the smelter companies to court to stop the worst aspect of the process, the smoking horror of heap roasting.

That action launched an environmental fight that lasted through the next decade, with ramifications that extended into the next century. Disenchantment with smoke pollution challenged the industry in Nevada, Utah, California, Arizona, and Colorado. Generations of industrial disregard for the environment came home to roost.

This issue was unusually difficult to resolve. Choosing profits over health, and vice versa, posed myriad complexities and conflicts. A resolution in favor of either could compromise a district's and a community's future. Health seekers, it was emphasized, were free to seek more agreeable locales to regain their vitality—and they did.

Meanwhile, doctors in the camps and towns "fought the good fight" in their attempt to provide competent health care for their patients. In the words of New York gubernatorial candidate Theodore Roosevelt, "We are face to face with our destiny and we must meet it with a high and resolute courage. For us is the life of action, of strenuous performance of duty; let us live in the harness, striving mightily; let us rather run the risk of wearing out than rusting out."

Very few mining community doctors rusted out. The best were remembered fondly. Butte doctors John Gunn, O'Dillon B. Whitford, and Joseph Tremblay were described as "loved and efficient." Arizona and Utah's Adolphus Noon, a former British Army veteran, and Deadwood's "dignified Prussian," Dr. H. von Wedelstaedt, who belonged to the Chinese masons, were equally revered. Estelline Bennett lovingly recalled von Wedelstaedt and his kindness. Her tribute to him stands for them all: "[He carried] a personal interest not only in our health, for which he felt entirely responsible, but in our general welfare no less."[12]

As the century came to a close, the rushes of 1849 and 1859 seemed long past. Because of their urban and cosmopolitan situation, residents of the mining communities had found their medical care much closer at hand and more varied than that received by the average rural westerner. In terms of health conditions, their predicament was little different from that in the East, where the major infectious epidemics had claimed at least as many lives as they had in the West. Life expectancy was short and infant mortality high everywhere.

California in 1849–1850 exhibited deadly extremes of disease and sickness unequaled by any other western mining region. Major medical advances made inroads slowly in most mining regions, especially after they went into decline. The mining West contributed little advancement to the medical profession or to the improvement of treatments. It contributed instead to the spread of that "dark countercurrent of Westward expansion," opium smoking. Westerners recognized the opium problem early; Virginia City, Nevada, passed an ordinance against opium smoking as early as 1876. Enforcement proved to be the stumbling block.[13]

Nonetheless, mining community residents, particularly in the more primitive towns, were fortunate to have physicians and facilities available to them at all. Mining camps never stopped struggling to attract and keep doctors; neither did the western farming hamlets. Urban environments had drawbacks, too. Epidemics took hold more readily there than on isolated farms and mines. It was both the best and the worst of times, as popular English novelist Charles Dickens wrote.

Notes

1. W. A. Goulder, *Reminiscences of a Pioneer* (Boise: Timothy Regan, 1909), 233; Miller cited in Andrew F. Rolle, ed., *The Road to Virginia City* (Norman: University of Oklahoma Press, 1960), 73, 76, 90, 102; *Black Hills Pioneer*, August 12, 1876, March 7, 1879; Hughes cited in Agnes Wright Spring, *Pioneer Years in the Black Hills* (Glendale: Arthur H. Clark, 1957), 324–335; Paul Phillips, *Medicine in the Making of Montana* (Missoula: Montana State University Press, 1962), chapter 6; Estelline Bennett, *Old Deadwood Days* (New York: Charles Scribner's Sons, 1935), 179, 223, 277; *The Herald* (Silver City, New Mexico), January 20–March 17, 1877; *Park Record* (Park City, Utah), November 12, 1881; Lola M. Homsher, ed., *South Pass, 1868* (Lincoln: University of Nebraska Press, 1960), 77, 81, 91, 94, 109, 160; *Silver Reef Miner*, June 28, 1879, February 14, 1880; George W. Parsons, *The Private Journal of George Whitwell Parsons* (Phoenix: Arizona Statewide Archival and Records Project, 1939), 128–138. For a general overview of mining in these states, see William Greever, *The Bonanza West* (Norman: University of Oklahoma Press, 1963).

2. *Owyhee Avalanche*, May 19, 1866; *Black Hills Pioneer*, May 26, 1877; *Pinal Drill*, May 28, 1881; *Butte City Union*, November 4, 1883; *Park Record*, June 5, 1880, July 15, 1882; *Arizona Silver Belt*, October 25, 1879; *Black Hills Weekly Times*, April 6, 1878; *Silver Reef Miner*, April 12, May 21, July 9, 1879; Parsons, *Journal*, 265.

3. Charles M. Clark, *A Trip to Pike's Peak* (San Jose: Talisman, 1958 reprint), 17; Louisa B. Clapp, *Shirley Letters* (New York: Alfred A. Knopf, 1970 reprint), 47; Elliott West, *Growing Up With the Country* (Albuquerque: University of New Mexico Press, 1989), 217–219, 222, 229–231, 233; Foote cited in Roman Paul, ed., *A Victorian Gentlewoman* (San Marino: Huntington Library, 1972), 166–168, 198.

4. *The New American Family Physician* (Chicago: Geo. M. Hill, 1901 rev. ed.), 179–181, 230–234, 1040, 1067–1075, 1124; West, *Growing Up*, 225, 230–234; Frances E. Quebbeman, *Medicine in Territorial Arizona* (Phoenix: Arizona Historical Foundation, 1966), 154, 157, 166–167; John T. Waldorf, *A Kid on the Comstock* (Palo Alto: American West, 1970), 50; Dan De Quille [William Wright], *History of the Big Bonanza* (Hartford: American Publishing, 1877), 216; Bennett, *Old Deadwood Days*, 4–5; Mabel Barbee Lee, *Cripple Creek Days* (Garden City: Doubleday, 1958), 20; C. L. Sonnichsen, ed., *Morris B. Parker's White Oaks* (Tucson: University of Arizona Press, 1971), 36; Eliot Lord, *Comstock Mining* (Berkeley: Howell-North, 1959 reprint), 375.

5. Ballou cited in Christiane Fischer, ed., *Let Them Speak for Themselves* (Hamden, Conn.: Archon, 1977), 44; West, *Growing Up*, 225–226; Julie Roy Jeffrey, *Frontier Women* (New York: Hill and Wang, 1979), 69; Mary Melcher, "Women's Matters," *Montana* (Spring 1991), 47, 52, 56; Sylvia D. Hoffert, "Childbearing on the Trans-Mississippi Frontier, 1830–1900," *Western Historical Quarterly* (August 1991), 273, 276–279; Joseph B. Cooke, *A Nurse's Handbook of Obstetrics* (Philadelphia: J. B. Lippincott, 1904), chapters viii, xxvi; Susanna Townsend letters quoted in JoAnn Levy, *They Saw the Elephant* (Hamden, Conn.: Archon, 1990), 74–76, 236; Sandra L. Myres, *Westering Women and the Frontier Experience 1800–1915* (Albuquerque: University of New Mexico Press, 1982), 156, 266.

6. Mary H. Foote to Helena Gilder, December 7, 21, 1876, Huntington Library, San Marino, California; Melcher, "Women's Matters," 50; Hoffert, "Childbearing," 274–275; Myres, *Westering*, 154; Alvin Chase, *Dr. Chase's Recipes* (Ann Arbor: Author, 1864), 214; *New American Family Physician*, 917–949; Elizabeth Jameson, "Women as Workers," in Susan Armitage and Elizabeth Jameson, eds., *The Women's West* (Norman: University of Oklahoma Press, 1987), 151–152.

7. Melcher, "Women's Matters," 50; Jeffrey, *Frontier Women*, 58; Kenneth Ludmerer, *Learning to Heal* (Baltimore: Johns Hopkins University Press, 1985), 14; Myres, *Westering*, 155–156; T. J. Ritter, *The People's Home Medical Book* (Cleveland: R. C. Barnum, 1910), 389; *American Family Physician*, 921, 927; *Territorial Enterprise*, September 12, 1874.

8. Anne M. Butler, *Daughters of Joy, Sisters of Misery* (Urbana: University of Illinois Press, 1985), 67–68; *Mountain Democrat* (Placerville, California), April 22, 1854; Walter Van Tillburg Clark, ed., *Journals of Alfred Doten* (Reno: University of Nevada Press, 1973), v. 2, 867; Lee L. Stone, ed., *Sex Searchlights and Sane Sex Ethics* (Chicago: Science Publishing, 1922), 307; David Courtwright, "Opiate Addiction in the American West, 1850–1920," in *Medicine in the West* (Manhattan: Sunflower University Press, 1982), 23–24, 26–29; Henry O. Whiteside, "The Drug Habit in Nineteenth-Century Colorado," *Colorado Magazine* (Winter 1978), 49, 54, 59, 61–63, 65; *Great Southwest* (Durango, Colorado), October 26, 1892, December 25, 1893.

9. Whiteside, "The Drug Habit," 55, 59, 61–63; *Rocky Mountain News*, January 13, 1881; Clark, ed., *Journals*, v. 2, 868; Chase, *Dr. Chase*, 75; Bennett, *Old Deadwood Days*, 279; Ron James and Elizabeth Raymond, *Comstock Women* (Reno: University of Nevada Press, 1998), chapter 5.

10. *Seventh Biennial Report of the Bureau of Labor Statistics 1899–1900* (Denver: Smith-Brooks, 1900), 268–269; Quebbeman, *Medicine in Territorial Arizona*, 58, 222–223, 295; Lord, *Comstock Mining*, 374; Jake W. Spidle Jr., *Doctors of Medicine in New Mexico* (Albuquerque: University of New Mexico Press, 1986), 32–34, 41–44; Charles Denison, *Rocky Mountain Health Resorts* (Boston: Houghton Mifflin, 1881), xii; S. Anna Gordon, *Camping in Colorado* (New York: Authors' Publishing, 1879), 67–68; *Herald* (Silver City), April 22, 1876.

11. Sargeant to James G. Hague, January 22, 1899, Hague Collection, Huntington Library, San Marino, California; Montana, *Proceedings and Debates of the Constitutional Convention* (Helena: State Publishing, 1920), 754; *Bute Miner* cited in Donald Macmillan, "A History of the Struggle to Abate Air Pollution From Copper Smelters of the Far West, 1885–1933," Ph.D. diss., University of Montana, 1973, 16, 21–22; *Engineering and Mining Journal*, December 20, 27, 1890, January 24, 1891. See also Clark cited in Duane A. Smith, *Mining America* (Lawrence: University Press of Kansas, 1987).

12. *Respectfully Quoted* (Washington, D.C.: Library of Congress, 1989), 4; *Copper Camp* (New York: Hastings House, 1943), 138; Quebbeman, *Medicine in Territorial Arizona*, 118–119; Phillips, *Medicine in the Making of Montana*, 113, 114–118, 247–248; Bennett, *Old Deadwood Days*, 30–31.

13. Courtwright, "Opiate Addiction," 23, 28–29; John Duffy, "Medicine in the West," in James Breeden, ed., *Medicine in the West* (Manhattan, Kan.: Sunflower University Press, 1962), 5, 10; Phyllis M. Japp, "Pioneer Medicines," in *Medicine in the West*, 16.

7

"The Accident Is One of Those That Seem Inevitable in Mining"

MEDICAL PRACTICES AND DIAGNOSES IN TRANSITION

T HE EARLY MEDICAL EXPERIENCES OF MINERS in California and Colorado occurred time and again in the development of new mining operations in the states and territories west of the Mississippi River. The most important transformations were linked to new medical procedures and a greater consciousness of sanitation and public health. As mining branched out across the American West, miners everywhere experienced the same dangers and disabilities first associated with mining in California, Nevada, and Colorado. These earlier western excitements provided a training ground for both the workers and managers on subsequent mining operations. By the early twentieth century their positions of leadership in mining would be displaced by the copper trio—Montana, Utah, and Arizona. These new-comers as well as Idaho, South Dakota, New Mexico, and Wyoming shared a common mining heritage; their workers experienced the same dangers underground or in the mills and smelters. They attracted the attention of international investors and drew immigrants from around the world; their technological prowess excited the world and drew the curious from near and far.

Paradoxically, however, the region made few contributions to the development of medical science. Although mining companies might hire the most recent graduates of medical schools, the physicians went west into a medical wilderness. In a period when medical research and treatment experienced the same startling breakthroughs miners associated with mining, the work almost always occurred in metropolitan centers and initially those in Europe.

U.S. medical practitioners drew upon the new research of their Euro-pean mentors—Pasteur, Lister, Koch, and others who transformed age-old practices and assumptions within a mere quarter century. Not surprisingly, the technological developments in mining occurred at remote locations where new mineral resources were discovered and exploited scientifically.

Precisely the same phenomenon occurred in medicine, except that its resources were dense conglomerations of humanity that permitted the easy transmission of disease and aggregated opportunities for accidents. This is the reason Americans made important mid-century contributions to surgery, the treatment of wounds, the care of the injured, and the organization of medical personnel. For medicine the American Civil War was analogous to the rich deposits of copper found in Bisbee, Jerome, Bingham Canyon, or Butte or the new deposits of gold and silver in Coeur d'Alene and the Black Hills. The U.S. struggle entangled more humans in furious endeavor to do harm to one another than any event between the Napoleonic wars at the beginning of the nineteenth century and the Great War that began in 1914.

The creation of the U.S. Sanitary Commission during the Civil War created heightened consciousness about public health and sanitation. In 1872 supporters of these issues created the then controversial American Public Health Association (APHA), which briefly rekindled interest in sanitation and medical research. Although the APHA survived, its sanitary focus necessarily brought it into conflict with the quarantine-focused United States Marine Hospital. Seven years later Congress created a national health board, which was authorized to investigate, advise, and quarantine. Under the leadership of Dr. John S. Billings of the army medical service, the national health board began to gather vital statistics and other information that would eventually assist public health officials, but the organization itself expired when reauthorization efforts failed in 1883. Concerns with public health issues invariably attracted physicians and laymen with interests in engineering, statistics, and social reform.[1] Their collective concern with cleanliness and statistical analysis formed an essential element in the dramatic improvements that occurred in the late nineteenth and early twentieth centuries, but by the 1870s new discoveries in the study of bacteria transformed the ways in which medical practitioners addressed the causes of disease.[2]

Throughout the first half of the nineteenth century physicians and biologists had hypothesized and discussed the possible relationship between diseases and microscopic organisms, but the research on fermentation by French chemist Louis Pasteur conclusively established the link between microscopic organisms and the process of fermentation. Joseph Lister built upon Pasteur's work by reasoning that such organisms caused putrefaction in wounds, just as they caused molds and fermentation. Using carbolic acid mist in operations and sterilization of hands and instruments, Lister eliminated bacterial infections and promoted physical healing. During the next two decades U.S. physicians gradually adopted Lister's procedures and thereby made new surgery both possible and practical.[3]

In 1876 Robert Koch proved that the anthrax bacillus produced anthrax. Building upon the earlier work of Casimer Davaine, Koch isolated
pure cultures of anthrax, injected it into healthy animals, and recovered
anthrax bacilli from the blood of the then sick animals. Nearly simultaneously, Pasteur completed identical research that demonstrated conclusively
the link between a particular microorganism and a particular disease. Koch's
new contribution was the development of the solid cultural medium,
which permitted him to isolate the anthrax bacteria and prove its singular
role in the transmission of the disease to healthy animals. By 1882 Koch's
technique became generally known and thereafter widely employed. In
that same year he reported that he had isolated the microbe that caused
tuberculosis, yet it required another decade before U.S. laboratories were
established simultaneously in Philadelphia and New York City.[4] Between
the late 1870s and 1905 the bacteriologists discovered the microbes causing
tuberculosis, cholera, gonorrhea, pneumonia, diphtheria, typhoid, tetanus,
bubonic plague, and syphilis. These discoveries originating with Pasteur's
proof of bacterial fermentation in 1858, the dramatic confirmations of
bacterial infections by Pasteur and Koch, and the emergence of medical
laboratories in 1892 paralleled the nineteenth-century phases of the western
U.S. mining industry.

Gradually, insights gained from Pasteur and Koch altered U.S. medical
training and were applied to the medical hazards found in both mining
communities and mines. Here miners lived in close proximity to other
individuals and worked in a hazardous and unsanitary environment for
eight to twelve hours daily. Numerous commentators describe miners
making friends with rats and mice—their companions in the underground
solitude and transmitters of dread diseases. Large mines often used horses
and mules for haulage, and they, too, posed problems for sanitation—their
offal joined human excrement and spit as sources for disease and ill odors.
As late-nineteenth- and early-twentieth-century medical researchers made
undisputed progress in the diagnosis and treatment of diseases, doctors
began to identify practices and procedures that clearly improved health or
chances of recovery from illness, accident, or injury.[5]

Similarly, improvements in sanitation began to create a healthier environment wherever people congregated in groups. Richard Shryock described
the remarkable success of improved sanitation in reducing the prevalence
of typhus fever in England, where there had been 885 deaths per million
people in the mid-nineteenth century and only 3 per million by the 1890s:
"This continued improvement occurred before any rational knowledge of
either cause or carrier was attained." The culprits in the transmission of
the disease were body lice, although this was not accurately theorized until
1909. Other insect-transmitted diseases included Rocky Mountain spotted

fever and bubonic plague. Similarly, wars proved vehicles for verifying the effectiveness of certain procedures. The Franco-Prussian War served as a controlled experiment on the effectiveness of vaccination against smallpox. The Germans had vaccinated their entire army and lost fewer than 300 men to smallpox, whereas the unprotected French Army lost more than 20,000 troops to death by smallpox. Similar progress was obtained in reducing cholera and typhoid when public water supplies were improved according to the recommendations of sanitary engineers.[6]

These scientific and procedural changes were strengthened by renewed interest in licensing physicians. Although the movement owed part of its inspiration to the effort to control medical schools' expansion in the 1870s, neither medical licensure nor the improvement of medical education had undergone profound changes before the last years of the nineteenth century. Similarly, the ratio of medical practitioners to American Medical Association (AMA) members around the turn of the century was 4 to 1 in Colorado, 9 to 1 in Montana, and 13 to 1 in California. Although a striking contrast to the current situation, the ratio of physicians in western mining states compared favorably with the situation elsewhere in the United States.

By the turn of the century the AMA was on the verge of reorganizing the U.S. medical community in a strategy that established the county medical society as the source of membership in the AMA hierarchy. This reform and a subsequent modification of the physician's code of ethics affirmed broad ethical principles rather than a prescribed set of rules. In the years after 1903 the AMA assumed primary responsibility for improved standards of medical education and endorsed Abraham Flexner's investigations of American medical schools. The publication in 1910 of the *Flexner Report*, which identified specific deficiencies in medical education, and work on the proper functions of local medical associations by AMA organizer Joseph N. McCormack, helped establish the AMA as both an advocate for improved medical education and an interrelated organization of physicians.[7]

These developments in medical practice and among medical practitioners had an important impact on the changing character of the treatment available to miners, their families, and their communities. The character of mining accidents and ailments changed little in the late nineteenth and early twentieth centuries when mining expanded into the other important western states and territories: Missouri, Montana, Idaho, South Dakota, Utah, New Mexico, and Arizona. Throughout this region the accelerated pace of industrialization and the attendant changes in mining labor continued to make mining the most hazardous occupation in the United States. As mines grew deeper and more mechanized, the causes of underground injuries remained those that had afflicted the early Californians, Nevadans, and Coloradans—namely, falling rock, explosives, and miners' falls.

Fatality rates among miners remained between 3.1 and 3.8 deaths per 1,000 employees. According to Alan Derickson, this fatality rate was 10 times higher than that among comparable manufacturing occupations. According to the U.S. Bureau of Mines, 357,299 nonfatal accidents occurred between 1911 and 1920, which meant that on average more than 20 percent of the typical workforce in a mine suffered injury each year. There is no reason to suspect that similar statistics had not prevailed during the last third of the nineteenth century.[8]

As industrial development spurred the rapid implementation of air drills and deeper mining, miner's consumption, or silicosis, grew in importance as an occupational disease among western metal miners. In the expanding industrial regimen, power drills, rapid development, and improved explosives were the contributing aspects of mine labor that put more dust, hence more free silica, into the underground environment. As Derickson pointed out, the pace of the mining and the depth of the work also accelerated with the new technologies, thus forcing miners to breathe both more rapidly and more deeply. This created a situation in which the probable danger from silicosis increased dramatically in the late nineteenth century.[9]

Miners recognized the dangers of their vocation and turned increasingly to mutual aid to ameliorate their discomforts, accidents, and diseases. From their inception miners' unions had focused on care of injured or sick comrades because of the nature of mining and the overwhelmingly male character of western mining in these years. In communities where men customarily outnumbered women and where family men were less common than bachelors, miners had to devise ways to take care of themselves and their own. The alternative for sick or injured miners was the county or community poorhouse—the U.S. alternative for persons without relatives or those unable to care for themselves. These institutions were universally scorned by contemporaries. One went to the "poor farm" when there were no alternatives. Unfortunately for critically injured or chronically ill miners without families, they could easily find themselves in this situation.[10]

Since miners suffered recurrent injuries and an as yet little understood occupational disease in their chosen vocation, they turned inward to avoid both the inferior treatment and the ignominy accorded those dependent on the poorhouse or county hospital. The earliest unions had taken responsibility for their injured or ill brethren. Local unions customarily provided their members with temporary assistance from the "sick committee," a modest weekly stipend during convalescence and death benefits when needed. The various early unions and their successor, the late-nineteenth-century Western Federation of Miners (WFM), continually struggled with the implications of aiding their sick and wounded colleagues. Developments in Idaho, Montana, and South Dakota made these emerging mining states early centers of union activity. Independent unions and WFM locals took distinctive action to provide assistance for those in need of medical attention. For example, turn-of-the-century locals in DeLamar, Idaho, and Terry, South Dakota, hired their own doctors, who were expected to treat injured miners. The locals took this action both to control the costs of medical assistance and to provide reliable health care for their membership.[11]

The purposes of mutual aid were both broader and more self-interested, according to Derickson. He contends that the establishment of union-sponsored medical assistance aided with recruitment, provided an alternative to wage increases or hours reductions, assisted members during national or regional financial adversity, served as a conservative outreach program to attract men reluctant to affiliate with a radical group, overcame racial and ethnic tensions that characterized the mining workforce, and projected a cooperative and generous image within communities often dominated by individualist, capitalistic, and exploitative absentee owners and corporations. Symptomatic of this communitarian and cooperative aspiration, the Butte Miners' Union proclaimed in 1913 that all of its members extending back thirty-five years had been buried with proper respect and ceremony.[12]

The work-related complications miners encountered in states and territories other than California, Nevada, and Colorado were identical to those miners first encountered in the earlier mining communities. One notable exception was the situation in Delamar, Nevada, which gained an early reputation as one of the most dangerous operations in the West. Indeed, the situation at Delamar confirmed for many the probable dangers mine dust posed for those who worked in it over a prolonged period. In Delamar the initial mill crushers engaged in dry crushing and emitted the silica and quartz particles directly into the air, which carried this rock dust downwind to cover the lower end of the community. Because the prevailing winds carried the quartz debris over the village itself, Delamar became a dreaded camp where both miners and their families suffered from the "Delamar fever." The disease was so widespread in the population that in the early fall of 1895 residents were ordered to clean up their properties and to boil water because community and company leaders suspected a form of cholera was causing the widespread affliction of miners and their families.

By 1899 the mill dust was generally recognized as the source of the community's misery and death, but the company obdurately refused to modify its mills to reduce silica emissions. Although the mills were eventually and reluctantly fitted with filters, the situation underground did not change.

According to John Townley, former miners reported "a coating of white, talc-like dust" several inches deep throughout the mining operations. This underground environment was unquestionably one of the worst in the West because the fine particles were easily tracked from the mining faces throughout the underground workings, leaving all underground men susceptible to the dread "Delamar fever." The progression of this occupational disease was sure and, in this environment, relatively swift. First, the silica damaged the lung tissue, which provoked internal bleeding and lung lesions, followed by an agonizing death. Townley concluded that "often a man reported to work, then suffered a massive hemorrhage at the mouth and nose, and died within a few days or weeks."[13]

Normally the progression of silicosis was more gradual. For example, in 1917 W. Rowland Cox advised his New Mexico mine manager H. E. Wheelock to find alternative, lower-elevation surface work for Sam Northey, who was suffering from "miners' consumption." Although Cox's letter showed genuine concern for a firm's longtime faithful employee, he did remind Manager Wheelock that if Sam accepted this transfer to another operation, "he will not be paid anywhere near the money he is earning now, but . . . I think we owe him this consideration." Cripple Creek, Colorado's, Mabel Barbee Lee described her father's gradual and painful death from silicosis. As she became conscious that he had the dread disease, she remembered the painful symptoms that had transformed Jonce Barbee from a vigorous and proud miner and father into a physically broken man: "I found him slumped over a woodshed, gasping for breath. His face was drawn and pale. I took hold of his arm, trying to help him. 'I'm all right now,' he said, pushing me aside and making his way slowly into the yard. He walked with a stoop, his hands clasped behind his back, his eyes fixed on the ground as though still searching for the elusive float."[14]

When Jonce Barbee died in 1905, his daughter returned to Cripple Creek for his funeral and commented pathetically on the little he retained at the end of his life—an old fiddle, a pipe, a tablespoon, a partially consumed bottle of cough syrup, some letters, a broken pencil, a twenty dollar gold piece, and his Masonic watch chain. At the end he had sold his wife's beloved earrings and had spent the last of his money. The process had taken almost five agonizing years, a time period in which a vital laborer had become a pathetic invalid.[15]

In all probability Jonce Barbee died from either pulmonary tuberculosis or pneumonia, secondary infections to which silicosis often led. His death, alone in a boardinghouse, was not atypical. Some died in hospitals or in the company of friends; the deaths could be from peaceful "cardiorespiratory failure," but others died in violent and bloody coughing spells. For the Barbees the disease had been a source of shame. James C. Foster reported the similarly remarkable fact that only one miner, Dennis Sullivan, had ever sought direct assistance from the WFM conventions, and even more remarkably, his was one of only two references to miners' consumption between 1900 and 1920. Derickson concluded that most deaths from silicosis "were cursorily dismissed in newspaper reports." The occupational disease did not fit the mold of booster journalism and so was relegated to insignificance in the newspaper accounts of its victims. Since silicosis was often confused with tuberculosis or pneumonia, Derickson estimated that 20 percent (approximately 30,000 individuals) of early-twentieth-century metal miners suffered from the disease at any given time.[16]

Late-nineteenth-century physicians understood little about the causes of miners consumption and so could do little more than prescribe cough syrups, lower altitudes, and less strenuous lifestyles. Beginning with the Delamar incident and the nearly simultaneous diagnosis of the dread disease in Australia, Canada, and South Africa, public health officials turned increased attention on the disease and the circumstances that produced it. Tragically, silicosis was a preventible illness because it occurred only when microscopic particles of silica (0.5 to 5 microns in size) were taken into the lungs. Larger particles were screened out by the nasal cilia, and smaller particles were exhaled without complication. Furthermore, only dry drilling and blasting released these killing particles. Wet drilling and the use of respirators dramatically reduced the dangers from this deadly disease.[17]

Although miners and mine operators could not reach consensus on appropriate strategies for combatting miners' consumption, other underground hazards proved subject to remedy. For example, hoisting accidents had plagued the early Comstock miners. By the early twentieth century, haulage accidents had been dramatically reduced through local or statewide adoption of underground bell signals. Even Wyoming adopted mine signals, which combined to form a vital source of communication between hoisting engineers and subterranean workers. Why were bell signals adopted when mine sanitation remained a matter of choice? The partial explanation must include the fact that both management and miners had much to lose if haulage accidents continued. The Wyoming signals were adopted by C. E. Jamison, state geologist of Wyoming, and their posting was mandatory in the engine room and at each level or station underground.

SIGNALS
1 Bell—Hoist
1 Bell—Stop if in motion
2 Bells—Lower
3 Bells—Men on, run slow
7 Bells—Accident. Hoist or lower by verbal orders only
3-2-1 Bells—Ready to shoot.[18]

Most mining hazards continued without such careful regulation. Miners needed to develop their own sense of caution, both above and below ground. E. D. Gardner, an early-twentieth-century miner and later Bureau of Mines official, confided in his diary his concern about the danger associated with commuting to work on the aerial tram: "Yesterday when I was at the place the highest from the ground the tram stopped a few minutes and gave me a chance to look around. I saw if anything should go wrong anyone on the tram wouldn't have one chance in a hundred of getting off alive." One month later he reported that he encountered bad air underground and had also mishandled running a hoist, crashing it into the bottom of the shaft. Five years later Gardner wrote to his friend Joe Manwaring, who managed Utah's Parvenu Mine, and complimented him on work that improved the ventilation in the underground stopes. Gardner concluded: "You should be able to get the best miners in there now."[19]

Other miners and operators reported the same concerns for underground safety in mines in New Mexico and Arizona. New Mexican Ernest Le Neve Foster encouraged Jefferson Reynolds to consider installing a good mechanical exhaust and electrical haulage system underground to lessen the danger and loss of time associated with "bad air." Bad air, or unvented powder gas, killed careless miners in both New Mexico and Arizona, where men forgot to turn on the compressed air lines used to ventilate the underground workings. The New Mexican accident killed Jose R. Lopez, severely injured Jose Montes, and frightened Italian de Col Dominico when Montes entered the 400-foot level and was overcome by bad air. Lopez died in a rescue attempt that caused him to fall from a ladder to his death when he, too, was overcome by the poisonous gas. In Arizona two miners died when Agapito Guterriz encountered poisonous gas that killed both him and his rescuer, Charles Jenkins.[20]

Miscellaneous accident reports from the mines of Arizona, Utah, and New Mexico confirm the ease with which miners could be injured, permanently scarred, or even killed while working underground. John Brockman, manager of Barringer Mine, reported a fatal cage accident on March 26, 1903, when a pump man was hit in the B shaft. Several months later a man named Smith sustained serious injuries in the same mine when he was "fooling around with the framing machine," which threw a piece of wood back into his face, breaking his jawbone and severely cutting him. The accident report indicated that he would be permanently disfigured. In Utah's Bingham Canyon, Frank Crampton nearly lost his life while opening hung-up ore chutes, and New Mexico's Fanny Mine sustained two fatalities when cage tender Antonio Breto and pipe and track man Simon Tate were crushed by a load of drilling steel that became dislodged during transit to the surface. In the preceding year another man lost his life when he looked down into a shaft just as the cage was being lowered. In recounting the death of Guernsey Piper, A. J. Anderson concluded that although Piper was an experienced mine worker who understood ordinary safety procedures, "the accident is one of those that seem inevitable in mining."[21]

These accidents produced fatalities and injuries that were characteristic of mining in California, Nevada, and Colorado. In most instances the break-throughs in medicine had little impact on these unfortunate mine workers. Daniel M. Barringer's employee named Smith presumably recovered from the disfiguring wound to the head, which might have been fatal in earlier years. Almost certainly he was taken to the company physician who cleansed his wound and administered antiseptics that retarded bacterial infection. Those who died or succumbed to poisonous gases received treatment that would likely have changed little since the early days. Broken bodies and poisoned or damaged lungs still proved virtually impossible to treat. Soon improvements in rescue techniques, artificial respiration, and respirators would hold out more hope for men who encountered "bad air" and were alive when evacuated from the poisoned environment.

This chapter began with an admission that American medical practitioners contributed less to the nineteenth century's remarkable transformation of medical procedure, knowledge, and research than their European peers. Such innovation as occurred was normally remote from the mining regions of the American West; yet the U.S. enthusiasm for technological innovation quickly reversed this dependent relationship. During the first two decades of the twentieth century U.S. medical science laid the foundation for what became the most creative and transforming era in the history of medicine. This spectacular improvement in medical knowledge and practice quickly began to transform the treatment of injured or ill miners. In an era where technological innovation had permanently altered the character of miners' work, it is not surprising that it also transformed the character of health care. Medicine had changed as dramatically in half a century as had mining; camomile became as scarce as the arrastra and surgery for compound fractures as successful as the new open-pit mining at Bingham Canyon, Utah.

Notes

1. Richard Harrison Shryock, *The Development of Modern Medicine: An Interpretation of the Social and Scientific Factors Involved* (Madison: University of Wisconsin Press, 1979 [1936]), 240–245.
2. Shryock, *Development of Medicine*, 246.
3. Shryock, *Development of Medicine*, 277–281; William G. Rothstein, *American Physicians in the Nineteenth Century* (Baltimore: Johns Hopkins University Press, 1972), 255–257.
4. Shryock, *Development of Medicine*, 282–284; Rothstein, *American Physicians*, 263–265, 268–269.

5. Shryock, 304–314; Ronald C. Brown, *Hard-Rock Miners: The Intermountain West* (College Station: Texas A&M University Press, 1979), 40–41, 95.

6. Shryock, 319, 322–323.

7. James G. Burrow, AMA: *Voice of American Medicine* (Baltimore: Johns Hopkins University Press, 1963), 16–20, 27–44; Rothstein, *American Physicians*, 316–323.

8. Alan Derickson, *Workers' Health, Workers' Democracy: The Western Miners' Struggle, 1891–1925* (Ithaca: Cornell University Press, 1988), 36–39. See also Mark Wyman, *Hard-Rock Epic: Western Miners and the Industrial Revolution, 1860–1910* (Berkeley: University of California Press, 1979), 86–143; Brown, *Hard-Rock Miners*, 59, 66–69, 72–73, 76–77, U.S. Bureau of Mines cited on 175–176.

9. Derickson, *Workers' Health*, 39–41; quote, 39.

10. Derickson, *Workers' Health*, 61–63.

11. Derickson, *Workers' Health*, 63–72. Derickson's account of the medical assistance provided by WFM locals is a model study of union health care and the rationale that made it necessary in a U.S. society that was barely groping for means to ameliorate the impact of the rapid industrialization of the late nineteenth and early twentieth centuries.

12. Derickson, *Workers' Health*, 80–85.

13. John Townley, "The Delamar Boom," *Nevada Historical Society Quarterly* 15 (Spring 1972), 10-12; quote, 10.

14. W. Rowland Cox to H. E. Wheelock, January 11, 1917, Blumenthal Papers, Special Collections Department, Zimmerman Library, University of New Mexico, Albuquerque; Mabel Barbee Lee, *Cripple Creek Days* (New York: Doubleday, 1958), 62.

15. Lee, *Cripple Creek Days*, 68–70, 184, 220–222.

16. James C. Foster, "Western Miners and Silicosis: 'The Scourge of the Underground Toiler,' 1890–1943," *Industrial and Labor Relations Review* 37 (April 1984), 371; Derickson, *Workers' Health*, 48–52.

17. Foster, "Western Miners and Silicosis," 373–376.

18. C. E. Jamison, State Geologist of Wyoming, *Mineral Resources of Wyoming and the Mining Laws of the State and of the United States*, Bulletin 1, Series B (Cheyenne: [Wyoming State Geologist], 1911), 83–84.

19. Diary of E. D. Gardner, August 8, and September 4, 1907, Box 42; and copies, E. D. Gardner to Joe Manwaring, May 31, June 5, 1912, Box 39 in the E. D. Gardner Collection, American Heritage Center, University of Wyoming, Laramie.

20. Ernest Le Neve Foster to Jefferson Reynolds, October 17, 1912, in Letterbook, 1906–1912, 53, in Ernest Le Neve Foster Collection, Western History Department, Denver Public Library; A. J. Anderson to W. Rowland Cox, Consulting Engineer, July 15, 1914, Box 1, in the Blumenthal Collection, University of New Mexico, Albuquerque; "Report of Mine Inspector for Six Months Ending March 31, 1914," 1, in the Summary of Fatal Accidents, Arizona Copper Company Collection, University of Arizona, Tucson.

21. Copies, Daniel M. Barringer to John Brockman, and Barringer to R.A.F. Penrose Jr., April 2, 1903, and August 14, 1903, Correspondence December 30, 1902, to October 2, 1903, in the Daniel M. Barringer Collection, American Heritage Center, Laramie; Frank Crampton, *Deep Enough: A Working Stiff in the Western Mine Camps* (Denver: Sage, 1956), 85–87; A. J. Anderson to W. Rowland Cox, August 5, 1914, and December 22, 1913, Box 1 in Blumenthal Collection, University of New Mexico, Albuquerque.

8
"Fired With the Faith of Fools"
ALASKA, 1897–1910

I wanted the gold, and I sought it;
I scrabbled and mucked like a slave.
Was it famine or scurvy—I fought it;
I hurled my youth into a grave.

THUS DID ROBERT SERVICE capture the essence of the days of 1898 in these opening lines of "The Spell of the Yukon." The Klondike rush freely crossed international boundaries when both isolated Alaska and Canada's Yukon Territory became caught up in the excitement. Illness and disease knew no boundaries either, as they assaulted the rushers with both old and new plagues and problems.

As far back as the early 1880s, gold had been mined in small quantities in the upper Yukon River. The pace of discovery picked up in the 1890s, and soon the tiny mining camp of Yukon City had arisen to serve miners' needs. Then, in August 1896, George Washington Carmack made the major discovery on soon-to-be-named Bonanza Creek. He at least holds the primary claim to the honor. A yield of up to $800 from a single pan of pay dirt sparked the "snow-balling stampede" that gained poetic fame for Robert Service. Jack London, who portrayed the times in his short stories and novels, also enjoyed the rush's literary benefits. In "All Gold Canyon" London pictured what it was like to make a bonanza discovery: "It was only half rock he held in his hand. The other half was virgin gold. He dropped it into his pan and examined another piece. Little yellow was to be seen, but with his strong fingers he crumbled the rotten quartz away till both hands were filled with glowing yellow. . . . It was a treasure-hold."

It would take some time for the good news to travel south to the states, but when it reached them, Americans braced for yet another rush. The lure of gold drew the adventuresome and the greedy to Service's northern climes, which challenged them with treacherous ice and snow, bitter cold, and numbing darkness that lasted for months.

The first ships carrying gold docked in San Francisco and Portland in July 1897. "Show us the gold," cried watchers on the shore at Portland. The passengers had no trouble complying with the request—the ship carried at least 2 tons of it. The startling news flashed first throughout the country, then to the world. Canada and the United States were instantly infested with an epidemic of gold fever. Alaska presented the opportunity for one last adventure, another chance to test one's skill and luck against the uncertainties of a mining rush. The *San Francisco Chronicle* caught the essence of the obsession in its July 17 issue: "Working men quit their jobs and joined the procession for the long and tedious journey northward. . . . Not since the days of '49 . . . has there been such excitement in mining circles."[1]

Gold precipitated the frenzy, but it was abetted by the 1890s depression, which still held the country in its tenacious grip after four dismal years. Reaching the goldfields would not be easy. Hundreds of miles of sea and land had to be negotiated, and midsummer had already slipped away, with winter coming on fast. In Dawson, the mining town at the heart of the rush, old-timer Joe Ladue warned that with winter near at hand, "privation and suffering is always the rule and not the exception." He was right, but nothing could deter the demand for passage on northbound ships. One aspect of this rush that caught the attention of the press was the number of "women stampeders," including a much-publicized women's expedition. Demand for ship passenger tickets drove the price as high as $1,000 per ticket.

The U.S. press speculated throughout the summer and fall as to whether starvation faced those stampeding northward and if there was enough food in the Klondike. Unquestionably, the rushers would encounter conditions unknown to previous prospectors and miners. The obvious one was the harsh climate. Less obvious was the heavy involvement of Canadian government officials, including the ever-present Royal Canadian Mounties who would ride herd on the invaders. This would not be the typical freewheeling stampede once the rushers reached the Yukon Territory.

Seasickness, crowded conditions, and unpalatable food affected some rushers long before they reached Skagway, Nome, or whatever port they were headed for. When winter set in, all they could do was wait and worry about travel routes and trail conditions. The impatient ones who tried to reach the mines during the height of winter paid with their lives or their health. Their tragedies did not deter the others, who whiled away the time with dreams of fortunes. In the spring the rush of '98 began in earnest.

Reminiscent of 1849 and 1859, the Klondike rush of 1898 lured about 100,000 people to set out for Dawson; approximately one-third actually arrived. Most landed in Skagway or neighboring Dyea where their troubles began. They were forced to climb over steep, torturous, snow-covered Chilkoot or White Pass before sailing down the inland waterways through fierce rapids and hordes of voracious mosquitoes. The stress and strenuous labor took a terrible toll on lives and health. Analogous to 1849, an alternative all-water route existed that constituted 4,500 miles over the Pacific Ocean from Seattle. The Bering Sea and the Yukon River then brought the rushers to Dawson, although sometimes too late to tap the very short prospecting season.

The Klondike was a poor man's paradise for two or three seasons before companies took control and dredging slowly eradicated the physical evidence of earlier individual struggles. Fortunately for the rushers, the discovery of gold on the Seward Peninsula near Nome prompted a second rush in 1899–1900, allowing them to hold onto their dreams a little longer.[2]

A bittersweet account of the transportation problems and illnesses that bombarded the rushers appeared in the report of First Lt. John C. Cantwell. He commanded the U.S. revenue steamer *Nunivak* on the Yukon River in 1899–1901 and was ordered to inspect every "vessel engaged in traffic on the river." The *Nunivak* also enforced the law and provided assistance to vessels and individuals who suffered a "legitimate case of distress." Overburdened and less than river-worthy boats and rafts crowded the waterways during the navigation season. Some prospectors made their way along the banks, traveling by dog teams or simply walking to a new discovery. "Destitute or in distress" individuals were taken onboard the *Nunivak*; the rest were required to make their own way. Mosquitoes and swarms of "minute gnats" bedeviled everyone indiscriminately.

An epidemic of smallpox in July 1900 kept Cantwell and his crew on duty at St. Michael, at the mouth of the Yukon River. The government imposed a quarantine to prevent the disease from spreading up the river. Cantwell concurred that "once in the river its progress through the country would be like wildfire." A detention camp was organized on Egg Island, "some 10 or 12 miles from St. Michael," and all mail was taken onboard the *Nunivak* and fumigated. By the twenty-fourth, with all danger past, the quarantine was lifted.

The rushers were not the only ones to succumb to illness. An epidemic of measles struck the natives in the region and ravaged their settlements when pneumonia combined with it. As the steamer pushed up the river, the crew observed firsthand the horror of villages with barely anyone well enough to fish or hunt. Many sick and starving people were "simply dying like flies." The ship's doctor and crew gave what aid and comfort they could with their available medicine and supplies.

For the first time since 1848–1849, scurvy plagued the rushers. An 1890 government report vividly described the "dreaded scourge" as it engulfed miners in the Copper River Valley. At Valdez the government relief expedition found some victims. Cabins were packed with unwashed, ill miners, "like sardines in a box":

> Most of them were more or less afflicted with scurvy, while not a few of them had frost-bitten hands, faces, and feet. . . . The odor emanating from these articles of clothing, the sore feet of those who were frozen, and the saliva and breath of those afflicted with scurvy gave forth a stench that was simply poisonous as well as sickening to a man in good health, and sure death to one in ill-health.

Cabins were at once appropriated for a hospital and a cookhouse, and "a crew [was] employed to run both places." Seventy-five more cases remained back in the valley—men too ill to make their way out.

Charles Brown, quartermaster's agent at Valdez, described the extent of the problem in his 1898–1899 report. In the short period of eight months, he had issued 9,675 rations to "the sick and destitute." Brown had also attempted to organize a relief expedition to Copper Valley during the winter, but snow, blizzards, and a dangerous glacier prevented them from reaching the sick. Then in March, medical supplies ran out just before Brown reported 277 additional cases of "destitute and scurvied people" the following month. The golden dream for many had become a black nightmare.[3]

Scurvy had broken out in Dawson even before Copper Valley's epidemic. Dr. J. J. Chambers, physician at Catholic Hospital, treated 40 mild cases in the spring of 1897. By winter the problem was worse, and he expected to "find 500 cases in Dawson and the Klondike district" by spring.

Dr. Leroy Townsend believed scurvy, "the most dreaded disease of the Alaskan prospector or miner," resulted from the insufficiency of fresh vegetables and the "long-continued use of salt and smoked meats," combined with the "use of stale or unwholesome food." Isolation, long winter-locked months, and high prices all contributed to dietary deficiencies. By now the cure (as well as the cause) for scurvy was known, but circumstances prevented implementation. Townsend noted that teas prepared locally by boiling young pine needles, the willow's inner bark, or juniper berries "have proven of value." Regarding the Copper River region, he pointedly observed that "considering the hardship and exposure undergone, it is surprising that so little sickness resulted."

Hardship characterized the life of prospectors/miners in the Yukon and Alaska. Many assumed their vigor and enthusiasm would ward off disease and that they would make it home with gold before being struck down. As in previous major gold rushes, guidebooks were published, the best of which tried to warn their readers of what lay ahead.

Placer Mining: A Handbook for Klondike and Other Miners and Prospectors appeared in 1897, and chapter 2 was entitled "How to Take Care of Yourself." A familiar item advised "all persons who contemplate going to the Klondike region to include in their outfits a medicine chest." Added to the fever pills, pain killers (morphine and opium), the old favorite quinine, laxatives, and salts was citric acid "in case of scurvy." The book rhapsodized over the health benefits of the North; life was longer, it claimed, "as residence is advanced from the equator towards the poles":

> For many constitutions the bracing effect of a trip to northern latitudes is positively beneficial. Snow and ice are not in themselves by any means injurious to the physical health of the average native of the temperate zone. They may be disagreeable, but they are not unhealthful.

The enthusiasm was qualified by this disclaimer: "To the weak, or those disposed to special ailments, conditions which are only invigorating to the man in average health are often absolutely fatal."

After concluding that "physical exhaustion, colds, scurvy, rheumatism, and snow blindness are the chief dangers . . . from a medical standpoint," the chapter dispensed some homey advice about camping and coping with life in the North. Included were such gems as how to handle a dog team, where to shoot a dog or horse ("if you have to"), and a warning not to "catch hold of the barrel [rifle] when 30 degrees below zero is registered." Experienced sourdoughs undoubtedly chuckled when they read parts of the book, but the author made a genuine effort to warn readers that only those equipped to handle hardship and arduous labor should go. How many heeded that warning is not known.[4]

Arthur Dietz was one of those who rushed north. Unquestionably, he met the standards recommended in *Placer Mining,* having been a YMCA physical activities director. Of his party of eighteen men, only four "reached civilization alive." Those four paid a terrible price to the Arctic sun: two were totally blinded, and the others were "left with very poor sight."

James Wickersham, a famous district judge and delegate to Congress, experienced severe snowblindness while on a late winter dogsled trip in 1901. He wrote in his diary, "My eyes feel as if they were filled with sand and I keep them covered with a bandage and hold on to the handle bars of the sled for guidance." He reached the mining camp of Circle, and with a day's rest and treatment, "my snow blindness disappeared." For those who neglected to wear their "goggles" or to otherwise protect their eyes, snowblindness posed a very real danger.

The usual treatment relied on using drops of a lubricating medicine for the eyes, then covering them and giving the patient some type of painkiller. A variety of home remedies was thought to help, including "pith of sassafras," elder flower tea, and laudanum. Miners in the states also experienced overexposure to the snow's glare, but its effects paled in comparison with those of the Arctic.[5]

Medical facilities were rare in the far North. Dawson reportedly had thirty "graduates of medicine" in November 1897, which placed it in the front ranks. Whether they all practiced their profession or had merely come north to mine is undetermined. The town did have a Catholic hospital, "a commodious log structure," with a capacity of fifty patients. The hospital charged $5 a day, with doctors' visits also $5, and provided a medical plan. For 3 ounces of gold paid annually, any Dawsonite could "be assured of free hospital quarters." *Harper's Weekly* correspondent Tappan Adney, who spent a winter in Dawson, concluded that "physicians did uncommonly well." He wrote: "A visit to the mines was sometimes as high as $500, the charge being regulated according to the 'victim's' ability to pay; and the price of drugs was proportionately high. One young doctor was said to have earned $1200 to $1500 a month." Doctors could prosper in the Klondike, as they had in other areas.

Dr. Chambers described the "prevailing disorders of the Klondike," besides scurvy. He mentioned "kidney troubles and mountain, or typo-malaria, fever." The latter revived memories of the 1849 overland parties and the plight of the 1859ers. He blamed the water of the Klondike and the Yukon, which "seems to possess chemical properties which act directly upon the kidneys as an irritant."

Another familiar sickness surfaced, the ubiquitous dysentery. Chambers estimated that in its mild form it afflicted 75 percent of the men "landing in Dawson." It usually yielded to treatment in a few days. Chambers himself came down with a bladder ailment, subsequently recovered, and continued treating patients at the hospital and in his office.

The ever-present danger of frostbite stalked all who challenged the north country. Survival entailed paying unwavering attention to protective measures. Clothing next to the skin froze very quickly when it became wet; a wet sock could cost a man a toe or worse. According to legend, Klondikers devised homemade gauges for determining the temperature. If a vial of rye whiskey froze, the sourdough smiled and went on his way. If a Perry Davis painkiller froze, he "dived back into his cabin." That elixir reportedly froze at –73° F.! Yet these hardy pioneers tolerated the abominable conditions, and Robert Service knew why. He wrote in the "Trail of Ninety-Eight":

Gold! We leapt from our benches. Gold!
We sprang from our stools.
Gold! We wheeled in the furrow,
fired with the faith of fools.

Newspaper accounts augmented the list of medical problems. Again, alcoholism multiplied the miners' woes and could be especially deadly in this climate. One story, headlined "Klondike Drinking Bout Kills Winner," confirmed that fact. The continued use of opium, laudanum, and morphine contributed to drug problems. Any of these could have led to "derangement," a commonly reported affliction. Isolation, cold, personal misfortune, and long winters all made an impact as well. Accidents, including accidental shootings, dog bites, bruising physical fights, and slipping on ice, as well as physical aliments like "la grippe," rheumatism, and colds, also affected the sourdoughs' health. An unusual episode in Nome in September 1909 involved the fear of an outbreak of "Siberian leprosy." Concern about leprosy had been mentioned elsewhere in the territory, so this incident was not isolated.[6]

The mouths of miners also exhibited problems. E. Hazard Wells, a man of the '97 rush, described Dawson dentistry that year: "There are four teeth-pulling artists in Dawson City, who charge $2.50 per jerk, balks not counted. An amalgam filling is inserted for $5." Miners of earlier years would have recognized the circumstances. Dentistry had not changed much, nor had the prices decreased. Too many patients still postponed a visit to the dentist until far too late for any cure but extraction.

Nonetheless, Dawson was the medical and dental hub for the entire district. For those who could get there, its facilities proved more than adequate. Those living in the outlying areas were ill served when distance and weather prevented easy arrival of a doctor or travel to the hospital.

Dr. Harry De Vighne described another familiar medical drawback of frontier medicine—the lack of rigid standards for practicing physicians:

> The only law in Alaska applicable to the healing art, enacted for the territory by an indifferent Congress but not even indifferently enforced, provided that to procure a license to treat the sick one must possess a diploma from a medical school and pay a five dollar recording fee. No one bothered to inquire whether the diploma was from a reputable institution, or whether it had been earned, bought, stolen, or in fact whether or not it was a medical diploma.

De Vighne ran across "one undaunted" practitioner whose sole credential "was an imposing looking certificate of membership in a lodge." The Mounties in Dawson tried to stem the tide by arresting as many "quacks" as they could and insisting that anyone who practiced procure a proper Canadian license. In U.S. territory medical free enterprise reigned.

De Vighne concluded logically and sadly that "as a result medicine in Alaska was represented by a variety of talent some of which was disreputable, and more of it decidedly questionable." Standards were better enforced in the states, although medical licensing did not become general until the 1890s. Even then, most licensing boards proved ineffective until well past the turn of the century, but up north in Alaska medical conditions were reminiscent of a generation earlier in the West.[7]

Richard Auzer recalled one man who explained that he did not have a license to practice medicine in the Klondike, but he would gladly give advice and do what he could to assist the miners. He placed a cigar box in a conspicuous place, along with a sign that read "Give what you can." Donations, Auzer claimed, "were liberal."

Old-fashioned remedies still ruled in some situations. One day a young man, "groaning with pain," appeared at the previously mentioned unlicensed man's office. The "doctor" examined him and announced that "he had contracted a disease from a woman, and he would try out a method of relieving his pain which was used during the Civil War when pain killers were unavailable." Obtaining a dozen packages of "Duke's Mixture," he proceeded to moisten the tobacco. The doctor applied it to "the swollen parts and in about a half-hour the man said the pain was easing." The satisfied patient soon left, "saying the treatment was a complete success." He placed five dollars in the contribution box. This patient was fortunate to find help nearby. Stories of lengthy dogsled trips to reach a doctor or hospital are part of the folklore of Alaskan mining.[8]

By 1905 newspapers and others were demanding regulation of doctors and territorial medical examiners. Times were changing on the last frontier. Laws were passed in 1908 and 1909, but lack of enforcement, as always, thwarted compliance. By then the opening era of Alaskan-Yukon mining had ended. Ahead lay a corporation-dominated industry, although prospectors would continue to search the frozen land for their own bonanzas. The last great rush was over. Once again home remedies and professional treatment had cured most rushers and settlers of their aches, pains, and myriad illnesses.

Notes

1. Robert Service, *The Best of Robert Service* (New York: Dodd, Mead, 1953), 1; Earle Labor et al., eds., *Short Stories of Jack London* (New York: Macmillan, 1990), 213; Melody Webb, *The Last Frontier* (Albuquerque: University of New Mexico Press, 1985), 77–81, 123–130; William Greever, *The Bonanza West* (Norman: University of Oklahoma Press, 1963), 332–338; T. H. Watkins, *Gold and Silver in the West* (Palo Alto: American West, 1971), 145–149; William R. Hunt, *Golden Places: The History of Alaska-Yukon Mining* (Anchorage: National Park Service, 1990), 20–24.
2. Ladue cited in Hunt, *Golden Places*, 24, 41–43, 72–73, 117–118; Greever, *The Bonanza West*, 338, 354, 361; Murray Morgan, *One Man's Gold Rush* (Seattle: University of Washington Press, 1967), 20–26, 43, 170–174.

3. John C. Cantwell, *Report of the Operations of the U.S. Revenue Steamer Nunivak* (Washington, D.C.: Government Printing Office, 1902), 59–62, 67–68, 69, 74; Brown cited in W. R. Abercrombie, *Alaska: 1899 Copper River Exploring Expedition* (Washington, D.C.: Government Printing Office, 1900), 14–15, 37, 39, 41.

4. E. Hazard Wells, *Magnificence and Misery* (Garden City: Doubleday, 1884), 130. Leroy Townsend's report is included in Abercrombie, *Alaska,* 44–47, which also cites Chambers. *Placer Mining: A Handbook for Klondike and Other Miners and Prospectors* (Scranton: n.p., 1897), 9–12; F. B. Smith, *The People's Health 1830–1910* (New York: Holmes and Meier, 1979), 197, 203–204, 244.

5. Arthur Arnold Dietz, *Mad Rush for Gold in Frozen North* (Los Angeles: Times-Mirror, 1914); I. James Wickersham, *Old Yukon* (Washington, D.C.: Washington Law Book, 1938), 76; T. J. Ritter, *The People's Home Medical Book* (Cleveland: R. C. Barnum, 1910), 242–244.

6. *Daily Gateway* (Seward), October 14, 1905; *Semi-Weekly Gateway* (Seward), January 27, 1906, January 5, March 9, 1907, October 1, 1908, May 2, September 11, 1909, February 5, May 28, 1910; Service, *The Best of Robert Service*; Charles Rosenberg, *The Care of Strangers* (New York: Basic, 1987), 237–241; Tappan Adney, *The Klondike Stampede* (New York: Harper and Brothers, 1900), 350; Mary Lee Davis, *Sourdough Gold* (Boston: W. A. Wilde, 1933), 131–135; *Today's Health* (February 1971), 10.

7. *Placer Mining,* 13–15; Wells, *Magnificence and Misery,* 130–132; Harry Carlos De Vighne, *The Time of My Life* (Anchorage: Alaska Northwest, 1984), 9; Davis, *Sourdough Gold,* 138–140; Robert Service, *Collected Poems of Robert Service* (New York: Dodd, Mead, 1940).

8. Richard Auzer, *Klondike Gold Rush* (New York: Pageant, 1959), chapters 1, 2.

9

"They May Yet Find Gold"

TIME OF RETRENCHMENT, 1900–1918

WITH THE NEW CENTURY CAME more corporation-dominated mining than ever before. The prospector and his faithful burro rode into the sunset, along with those who had followed him to the promising new strikes. A few more mining rushes, particularly in Nevada, electrified the public, but the time for the investor, the businessman, and the professional mining man had clearly arrived.

In Montana, Arizona, and Utah, copper mining surged ahead of the field with company towns, massive operations, and company control. Colorado's Cripple Creek and San Juan districts were still producing major quantities of gold and silver, but each had been mined for more than a decade and had settled into an industrial routine disturbed only by labor violence in 1903–1904. Coal became a stalwart of the new mining era; however, its nearly complete company control, ethnic workforce, and highly dangerous work conditions discouraged public attention and interest.

Small mining camps declined and disappeared as their discouraged residents moved to more promising locations. Throughout the West the "ghost towns" that dotted the landscape slowly crumbled back to the earth. Occasional visitors poked around, imagining what had taken place there in a West that now seemed as remote as the Civil War.

As the twentieth century matured, the mining West steadily lost its newsworthiness. Large companies, daily-wage miners, and corporation-dominated communities failed to ignite the urge to seek individual fortunes in a romantic land that lay to the west. Newspaper readers were all too familiar with the industrial-corporation story, which they could likely see unfolding in their own eastern and midwestern backyards. They turned to fresher, more current topics, and an era receded into history.

Many smaller mining camps found themselves devoid of doctors, who decamped along with most of their patients. Those who remained relied on themselves or physicians summoned from a nearby town. The telephone proved a great boon, but delays in a doctor's arrival were inevitable. The company towns supplied their own doctors, for whose services the miners generally paid with a monthly payroll deduction. The quality of services depended on the company's concern for its workers and the professionalism of the doctor it hired. The larger mining towns, such as Butte, Leadville, and Globe, continued to provide doctors and hospitals, although even there the number of practicing physicians varied with economic fortunes.

In this changing world of the twentieth-century West, Nevada was the home of the last of the great mining rushes. The Tonopah and Goldfield strikes of 1900 and 1904, respectively, brought thousands of would-be millionaires to the state, reviving its stagnant economy. The entire southwestern portion of Nevada found itself caught up in an old-time mining revival, with little camps and "promising" mines sprouting everywhere. Rhyolite typified them all. Platted in 1905, it soon evolved into a crude community of canvas and tent dwellings. Shortages of water and fuel did not deter the rushers, who converted the primitive surroundings into a town with wood and stone structures and a population of 6,000 in two years' time. One more time, one more rush. Far across mountains and deserts to the east, the Ely copper mines opened to furnish more economic incentives.

The silver and gold discoveries were new, but the problems that enveloped them were old. Deplorable sanitation conditions prevailed, with garbage scattered in the alleys and streets of towns and camps. Emmett Arnold, who settled in Goldfield in 1906, talked of the "grim specter" of what he called the "Black Death," pneumonia. A popular belief held that corpses of its victims turned black, therefore the name. It affected people of all ages and could be deadly in only a day or two. One doctor sadly admitted that no effective treatment for pneumonia was known, and "in the majority of cases, our best efforts result disastrously."

Three pneumonia outbreaks erupted in Goldfield during the 1904–1907 period. Frank Crampton, one of the fortunate survivors, wrote of the worst month—November 1906: "It was a humdinger and a lot of hard-rock stiffs, and stiffs, went over the hill to whatever reward they had coming to them." He himself grew steadily worse before his friends transferred him to Oakland because of overcrowded conditions in the Sacramento and Reno hospitals. Crampton recovered after a long convalescence to "get my strength back."

Arnold and Crampton were correct in their evaluations. Pneumonia proved the single greatest cause of death, accounting for over 33 percent of deaths in Goldfield during the boom years. One was reminded of the days of '49 when cholera had been the prevailing plague. The living conditions in both eras surely fueled the epidemics. Casual disregard for sanitary precautions also led to typhoid outbreaks, second only to pneumonia as a Goldfield killer.

State Board of Health physician Dr. S. L. Lee visited Tonopah to investigate the health situation there. He reported that seventeen had died of pneumonia in the first two weeks of 1902. Lee blamed the epidemic on the filthy conditions, a polluted water supply, and drinking festivities that marked the end of the year. Heavy consumption of alcohol created the usual complications. "Booze is cheap and flows like water," reported the *Goldfield Review* on November 16, 1907.[1]

Contagious diseases continued to be a constant threat during the boom periods in all these communities. Goldfield experienced a smallpox epidemic in the spring of 1904. Tragically, many residents seemed more intent on keeping the news from the outside world than in preventing its spread. A near panic consumed the community until the disease was brought under control.

The familiar story unfolded, one involving inadequate food and water supplies, lack of proper housing, a weak or nonexistent government organization, rapid population turnover, and little regard for health until an epidemic took hold. Californians, Montanans, and others would have recognized the scenario.

In most of these Nevada districts, water was at a premium. Rhyolite was able to find a solution to its scarcity because nearby springs allowed water to be piped into town. The wealth and fame of Tonopah and Goldfield attracted investors, who organized water companies to pipe water in or drill wells.

Marjorie Brown related her experiences at Tonopah. She purchased water once a week, "carefully using every bit" as she scrupulously conserved to meet all her household needs for drinking, bathing, and laundry. Raising a baby in Tonopah in 1905 demanded ingenuity. The lack of fresh milk prompted Marjorie to rear her children on malted milk; they "did pretty well." No pediatricians practiced in the community, so "we relied mostly on instinct and a trial-and-error method."

Despite the dearth of pediatricians, plenty of other doctors hung out their shingles in Tonopah (forty in 1907 alone). Most of them, Brown opined, appeared more interested in the illnesses and accidents of miners than in a general practice. Rumors about their character circulated rampantly. One "was whispered" to have been a drug addict in Alaska and subsequently had fled the "publicity of a murder trial," to which he was an accessory to the fact.

A "very charming English doctor" whom Brown remembered had an even more tragic life. This man lived in the community for several years before a scandal crashed in on him. He had left his wife in England for another woman, who was living with him at the time. His wife demanded a divorce and custody of his Tonopah son (by his common-law wife), heir to the title his father had also fled. The doctor refused her demands, and after the story became common knowledge, his "practice disappeared." Taking "refuge" in drugs only worsened his position, and he eventually left town.[2]

Anne Ellis also made it to Goldfield on her meandering trip throughout the mining West. Her experiences differed from Marjorie Brown's in the "mad but thrilling search for gold." Joy, her nine-year-old daughter, complained of what seemed a simple sore throat. "I have always been my own doctor, so now [I] do all the things I have formerly done," said Anne. Joy did not improve. When home remedies failed, Anne finally sent for a doctor who pronounced her daughter's illness diphtheria, "that dread word." The doctor prescribed antitoxin, which provoked this outburst: "I hate it—although it may save lives, it leaves many cripples, or did then." A cheerful child and "full of play," Joy died, although her sister Neita, also a victim, lived. Soon afterward Anne suffered a miscarriage that resulted from her "ceaseless round of work" and the stress of her family life.

Before the family returned to Colorado, Anne Ellis "borrowed" a white stone step from a schoolhouse under construction. It stood as Joy's headstone. Anne had earlier "cured" her husband of pneumonia by keeping Herbert "well plastered in onions." When he later succumbed to "spells," he appeared "gray and drawn" but continued to work, despite his illness: "We had the doctor, who did not know just what it was, but would give him a shot of morphine and leave." When the mines eventually began to close, the family left Goldfield, but this mother left part of her heart there: "So we leave, my greatest regret the little grave toward the west."

Anne Ellis's family medical problems and treatment could have been much the same at Angels Camp, South Pass City, or Alta anytime during the previous generation. Procedures had changed little, especially for the poor. A balanced diet was difficult to achieve for everyone except those who had money. Had she been able to afford them, Anne would have found in Tonopah's and Goldfield's finest restaurants the same elegant meals Virginia City and Leadville offered. Weather vanes of prosperity, the fancier restaurants began to close, signifying that decline was imminent.

A study of Goldfield's mortality rate in the years 1904–1909 found infectious diseases to be the primary killers. Respiratory diseases, tuberculosis, and other communicable diseases (typhoid and meningitis, for example) were responsible for half of the town's 779 deaths. Cancer, a rarity (although perhaps many cases went undiagnosed), accounted for less than 2 percent of the total, and cardiovascular and cerebrovascular diseases made up 9 percent. Women seemed more prone to tuberculosis than men and were seven times more likely to die of cancer. As mentioned previously, more Goldfield residents died of pneumonia than any other cause.[3]

Although women accounted for only 10 percent of Goldfield's deaths, their suicide rate soared to 37 percent of those who took their own lives.

Morphine, opium, and poison were the favorite methods. What created the depths of despair that contributed to this tragically high percentage cannot be ferreted from remaining records. Seemingly, there must have been added pressures on women from all walks of life compared with their sisters elsewhere, but the whys have been lost to history.

Older communities waged ongoing wars against the lack of sanitation and the prevalence of disease. As the tax base shrunk their problems multiplied; Leadville fell prey to a typhoid epidemic in the winter of 1903–1904. The State Board of Health came in to investigate, focusing particularly on the local water and milk supplies. "Careful investigation" finally cleared both, except private wells, polluted by a pattern of "marked sewerage contamination." Smaller camps, barely maintaining their existence, had even more troubles. Health ordinances were difficult or impossible to enforce; often the effort was simply abandoned. Health committees failed to function, and town councils seemed incapable of reversing the trend. Health matters lay far from the minds of St. Elmo's Board of Trustees, for example. The priority of this Colorado community was simply to find ways to prolong its life and that of its supporting mines. Much of the mining West now felt itself under the same pressures.

A few Colorado doctors, particularly some in the far western mining districts, encountered something previously unknown. It began with a small uranium rush, which opened mines and prompted reexamination of old dumps from Central City westward to Utah. A few miners in the uranium country west of Telluride subsequently experienced a strange type of "intractable" ulcer. A shrewd doctor soon discovered that the cause could be traced to carrying "choice bits of pitchblende" in their pockets. This habit was not unusual—miners and prospectors had always delighted in flaunting their specimens. They failed, however, to understand the strange characteristics of this new ore. These men received what today would be described as a radium burn.[4]

The personal heartaches that came, even after "modern medical advances," were no less traumatic to the individuals involved. Harriet Backus, who lived at Colorado's Tomboy Mine high above Telluride and later in Leadville, wrote about some of the tragedies in those places. Her best friend's young son died of meningitis, a neighbor gave birth to a stillborn baby, another friend left because of rheumatism aggravated by the high elevations, and Harriet's husband was seriously injured in a mining accident. She endured three successful pregnancies (one baby died soon after birth) and treated a rash of childhood illnesses.

As previously noted, in the first two decades of the twentieth century, the number of physicians in the mining communities declined. This trend reflected primarily the retrenchment in mining but also paralleled a general decrease of doctors in towns with populations under 5,000 throughout the country. The decline would worsen as the years went by. At the same time, better-trained physicians were coming out of medical schools. Medical research was improving, presaging the modern age of medicine. The young physicians showed a preference for larger cities, which offered better facilities, larger professional staffs, and higher incomes. Specialization became more popular and seemed more practical in urban centers. Most doctors in the mining West served as general practitioners whose schedules revolved around office hours and home visits.

Diagnostic procedures, prevention of infectious diseases, and surgical techniques continued to advance. With improved anesthesia, knowledge, and techniques, surgery was drastically transformed. Operations that had previously been impractical became easier and safer. Specific disease agents were being isolated, and the once major plagues of smallpox, diphtheria, tuberculosis, and the like were brought under some degree of control for the first time in world history. A heightened awareness of the importance of sanitary precautions improved both hospital and home treatments. The reading public, meanwhile, was becoming better informed about the benefits of improved medical science and practice, along with the significance of preventive medicine. Articles in magazines and newspapers brought news of the latest advances in the field.

The reputation of hospitals also improved. No longer seen as pest houses or death warrants, they were converted to havens for cures, childbirth, and surgical recovery. Better-trained nurses and staffs added to patient confidence. For the residents of most smaller mining communities, unfortunately, hospitals lay a day's or more journey from home.

Also unfortunate was the fact that advanced techniques and treatments migrated slowly to the mining West, especially after the recession hit all but a few districts. The most modern hospitals, specialists, and latest medical procedures could be found in regional centers such as Denver, Salt Lake City, and San Francisco, not in the once prosperous towns of Virginia City and Deadwood. Only Butte and a few other copper mining districts managed to maintain their prosperity up to 1914, when World War I shattered a decade of peace.[5]

World War I also marked an important turning point in western mining. Coal and base metals could contribute more to the war effort than precious metals, which continued to decline. Even in the last of the boom towns—Cripple Creek, Tonopah, and Goldfield—precious metals had become merely reminders of a bygone era by the time the United States entered the war in April 1917.

The end of the war brought no relief for the depressed mining communities. The inventions and innovations of a new age created no renewed prosperity for them. Automobiles, electric appliances, and other modern trappings invaded their streets, homes, and stores, but the abandoned and boarded-up buildings gave dramatic evidence of how far they had fallen. Yet these communities still constituted an important segment of U.S. society when the infamous and tragic 1918–1919 influenza epidemic struck with an impact not known before or since. It was first reported in the United States in March 1918, although its full impact awaited its deadly return in September of that year.

"Influenza and pneumonia" was ranked as the leading cause of death (11.3 percent of all deaths) in the United States at the turn of the century. Thus Americans were well aware of the potential dangers of the flu, whether living in a mining or a farming town. The "flu bug," even if called grippe, had been prevalent in mining communities since 1848, although the magnitude of the 1918–1919 epidemic was unprecedented.

Estimates start at 21 million victims worldwide. The flu killed over half a million in the United States and was particularly deadly at higher elevations; 7,783 Coloradans died within ten months. Misnamed "Spanish influenza" because of an early siege in that country, the flu probably originated in either the United States or China during the spring of 1918. Apparently, the epidemic was caused by a swine virus. It likely migrated to Europe, where it mutated into an even more deadly, virulent virus before finding its way back to North America in the fall. The fall and winter of 1918–1919 were the most devastating times, as two separate waves overran the country. Pneumonia frequently followed the flu, and the combination proved deadly. Doctors had little knowledge of the virus that caused influenza; many incorrectly attributed it to bacteria. They deduced correctly that it was a highly contagious airborne disease that flourished under crowded conditions. Nurse Bessie Finegan, who became one of its victims, remembered the epidemic clearly:

> It was awful. I was no sicker than the rest but I couldn't walk I was so weak. There was nobody on the streets that didn't have to go. Everybody on the street wore white surgical masks. I don't think it helped much, because everybody seemed to get the flu anyhow. . . . Two things happened to you. Suddenly you couldn't breathe, your lungs seemed to collapse, or else you hemorrhaged, and you hemorrhaged. There was nothing to do, the blood just gushed from your mouth and nose and you just died in a few minutes. Doctors got it. They didn't have nurses, even in the hospital the nurses were sick. So people, good people just volunteered.

Physicians seemed powerless. In desperation they tried quarantines and face masks, and people were warned to avoid crowds, to smother coughs, and to seek fresh air. Other recommendations made less sense, except to show the desperation of the times. Breathing deeply of "pure air," keeping a "clean heart," and avoiding tight clothes provided no protection. Nothing, it seemed, could stop the plague.

It seized the surviving Colorado mining camps and the more prosperous mining towns with equal vengeance. Theodore Drakulich, Angelina Sartore, and over 150 others died in Silverton—approximately 10 percent of this mountain-locked town's population. Silverton had the dubious distinction of having the highest percentage of residents die of any community in the country. Leadville had lost 223 residents when panicked grave diggers refused to handle any more bodies. "Strict and drastic" quarantine laws had no effect on the epidemic; it had to run its course.

St. Elmo's Board of Trustees bestirred themselves from a four-month hiatus to consider the flu crisis. "The mayor was requested to issue a proclamation establishing a quarantine" and to appoint a committee to ensure that the terms were carried out. The financially strapped government went so far as to hire a man, at a rate not to "exceed $1 per day," to enforce regulations. Long past its days of mining glory, Caribou, like St. Elmo, had no doctor. Home remedies—"sage tea, mustard plaster, onion poultices, and whiskey"—substituted for scientific measures. One man who felt himself coming down with the flu tried a "drastic cure"—a large dose of kerosene: "This made him temporarily very sick, but caused him to perspire so freely that he broke up the attack." Desperate conditions bred desperate measures, some of which worked as well as the best medical advice.[6]

Kerosene mixed with sugar or turpentine with honey had long constituted a folk remedy for a sore throat, so this attempted cure was not as astonishing as it might have appeared. In any case, most measures taken during the epidemic served only as palliatives.

The epidemic overwhelmed Colorado, and Montana, Alaska, and Nevada fared no better. Despite extraordinary precautions, the epidemic reached Nome and Skagway, then "ran like fire along a powder train" to Fairbanks, Copper Center, and other camps. The Yukon was successfully shielded until mid-April 1919. Native people suffered particularly hard in a land where serious illness in the harsh environment often meant death.

Butte and its surrounding county took every precaution but did not escape terrible suffering. Homes that harbored influenza cases were quarantined, causing the *Butte Miner* (December 6, 1918) to observe that confined children found no end of grief: "Nowhere to go but out, and nowhere to stay but in." The closing of public places and other spots where people congregated created resentment among some segments of the population. When the city allowed saloons to stay open, ministers protested. The county and city bickered over health regulations. Neither the disputes nor the restrictions served much purpose. The epidemic took a fearsome toll:

over 3,500 cases were reported in October, and 1,000 deaths occurred in the epidemic's worst six weeks.

Butte's smelter city, Anaconda, fared better. Anaconda boosters dusted off an old argument to explain the phenomenon. Local physicians believed gases spilling from the smelter killed the germs and explained the community's escape.

The flu silently crept into Nevada as well. It hit larger towns, such as Goldfield and Tonopah, and did not spare the rapidly ebbing mining camps. Pioche was actually given credit for instigating the last influenza wave in March 1919! Some communities tried quarantines, others banned public meetings. Ely placed a physician aboard a special car to treat train passengers who succumbed to the flu. Local remedies such as Indian root and sagebrush tea proved worthless. Cures were not to be had here or elsewhere.[7]

Inevitably, the great flu epidemic passed into the realm of history. The mining West and the rest of the country could turn to other matters in an attempt to put this tragedy far from their minds.

The race to El Dorado had ravaged its participants, whether in 1848 or 1918. The intervening generations had watched the settlement of the mining West, its exploitation, and the "busting" of most of its districts. Camps and towns had boomed, matured, and died, leaving behind mute evidence of their medical histories in cemeteries already crumbling. The survivors had lived out a dream, sometimes a nightmare, and lived to tell about it. Whether fortune rewarded their efforts, they still had "seen the elephant."

They had also witnessed a steady evolution of medicine and medical practices and the emergence of the modern age of medicine. Americans unquestionably could avail themselves of better medical treatment than that available before the Civil War. Drastic changes had already occurred, but they were nothing compared with the progress that would be made over the next fifty years. Precious few innovations had come from the West; the mining states had followed rather than led.

What these pioneers and later arrivals had experienced was hard to explain to contemporary Americans perched to enter the "roaring twenties." The western saga had joined the Civil War as part of America's past and was being replaced by the automobile, the Charleston, professional sports, and movies. Poet, writer, and westerner Thomas Hornsby Ferril described those bittersweet days in his poem "Magenta," set in Central City, Colorado. Whether in Fiddletown, California, in 1849 or in Butte, Montana, in 1918, the personal grief of mining life prevailed. No medical miracle could make a difference.

I spoke to Magenta of how the graves were sinking,
And Magenta said, "All this is tunneled under;
I think some of these ladies may yet find gold,
Perhaps," she sighed, "for crowns," and she continued:

"Maybe you never saw a miner dig
A grave for a woman he brought across the plains
To die at noon when she was sewing a dress
To make a mirror say she was somebody else."

"I never did," I said, and Magenta said:
"A miner would dig a grave with a pick and shovel
Often a little deeper than necessary,
And poising every shovelful of earth
An instant longer than if he were digging a grave,
And never complaining when he struck a rock;
Then he would finish, glad to have found no color."[8]

Notes

1. Russell R. Elliott, *Nevada's Twentieth-Century Mining Boom* (Reno: University of Nevada Press, 1966), 3–10, 47–48; Emmett L. Arnold, *Gold-Camp Drifter 1906–1910* (Reno: University of Nevada Press, 1973), 46; Frank Crampton, *Deep Enough* (Norman: University of Oklahoma Press, 1982), 47–48; Sally S. Zanjani, "To Die in Goldfield," *Western Historical Quarterly* (February 1990), 51–52, 53, 62–63; "Report of the State Board of Health, 1901–1902," *Appendix to Journals of the Senate and Assembly* (Carson City: State Printing Office, 1903), 5–7.

2. *Goldfield News*, May 6, 1904, January 6, 1905; Elliott, *Nevada's Twentieth-Century Mining Boom*, 48; Mrs. Hugh Brown, *Lady in Boomtown* (Palo Alto: American West, 1968), 53, 80.

3. Anne Ellis, *Life of an Ordinary Woman* (Lincoln: University of Nebraska Press, 1980 reprint), 248–254, 263–270, 277, 283–283; Henry J. Garrigues, *A Text-Book of the Diseases of Women* (Philadelphia: W. B. Saunders, 1901), parts 3, 6, 7; Joseph W. Conlin, *Bacon, Beans, and Galantines* (Reno: University of Nevada Press, 1986), 168, 194; Zanjani, "To Die in Goldfield," 49, 53–54; Henry O. Whiteside, *Menace in the West* (Denver: Colorado Historical Society, 1997), 20–30.

4. Zanjani, "To Die in Goldfield," 65–66; "Leadville Typhoid Epidemic," *Colorado Medicine* (February 1904), 151; St. Elmo Board of Trustee Minutes, July 1913–January 1915, Special Collections, Colorado College, Colorado Springs; Joseph N. Hall, *Tales of Pioneer Practice* (Denver: Carson, 1937), 51–52.

5. Harriet Fish Backus, *Tomboy Bride* (Boulder: Pruett, 1969), 61, 73, 108–109, 113–114, 244, 248–249; William Rothstein, *American Medical Schools* (New York: Oxford University Press, 1987), 67, 73, 119, 121–122; Kenneth Ludmerer, *Learning to Heal* (New York: Basic, 1985), 72–73, 75–78, 102; Brian Inglis, *A History of Medicine* (Cleveland: World, 1985), 144–145, 152, 154; Richard

Malmsheimer, "Doctors Only," in *The Evolution Image*, David Wetzel, ed. (New York: Greenwood, 1988), 28–29.

6. Stephen J. Leonard, "The 1918 Influenza Epidemic in Denver and Colorado," in *Essays and Monographs in Colorado History* (Denver: Colorado Historical Society, 1989), 1–2, 10; Rosemary Stevens, *In Sickness and in Wealth* (New York: Basic, 1989),101–102; James Cassedy, *Medicine in America* (Baltimore: Johns Hopkins University Press, 1981), 120–121; Monroe Lerner and Odin W. Anderson, *Health Progress in the United States 1900–1960* (Chicago: University of Chicago Press, 1963), 5, 11, 15; Pierce C. Mullen and Michael L. Nelson, "Montanans and 'the Most Peculiar Disease,'" *Montana* (Spring 1987), 50, 52; W.I.B. Beveridge, *Influenza: The Last Great Plague* (New York: Prodist, 1977), 30–33, 42–43; Bessie Finegan Interview, Durango, Colorado, January 5, 1976; Freda Peterson, *The Story of Hillside Cemetery* (Oklahoma City: n.p., 1989), vi; Rene Coquoz, *The History of Medicine in Leadville* (n.c.: n.p., 1967), 11, 14; St. Elmo Board of Trustees Meetings, June 4, 1918–February 4, 1919; *Boulder Camera*, January 24, 1944.

7. Phyllis Japp, "Pioneer Medicines," in James Breedam, ed., *Medicine in the West* (Manhattan, Kan.: Sunflower, 1982), 19; Alfred W. Crosby Jr., *Epidemic and Peace, 1918* (Westport, Conn.: Greenwood, 1976), 243–255; Mullen and Nelson, "Montanans," 54–55, 58, 60; *Butte Miner*, December 17–19, 26, 1918; Russell R. Elliott, "The Influenza Epidemic of 1918–1919," *Halcyon/1992*, 249–250, 253, 255–257.

8. Robert Baron et al., eds., *Thomas Hornsby Ferril and the American West* (Golden, Colo.: Fulcrum, 1996), 54.

10

"The Secret of Safety Work Is One of Leading People to Think"

MEDICINE IN THE MINES IN THE TWENTIETH CENTURY

ALTHOUGH COMMUNITY MEDICINE CONTINUED TO LAG behind the treatment accorded the ill in metropolitan centers here and abroad, the situation underground began to improve. The reasons for this phenomenon varied, but important aspects of the changes can be attributed to the growing curiosity of urban physicians and the occasionally combined interests of workers and management. If there was a single harbinger of the changes to come, William Henry Welch's selection in 1893 as dean of the newly created Johns Hopkins Medical School may have been that sign. In his initial address that proclaimed his visions for the school, he noted that Johns Hopkins would have a thoroughly scientific approach to medicine; the cornerstones were the laboratory, the clinic, and the hospital ward. In and of itself this was an important new direction for an as yet unorganized institution, but he went further. He proclaimed that the laboratory at Johns Hopkins would concentrate on social medicine; Hopkins physicians would pay special attention to such phenomena as housing, sewage, and work conditions. He later argued that the purpose of a medical education was "the training of young men and *women* [emphasis added] for careers of usefulness in the relief of human suffering and in the promotion of the general welfare."[1]

Welch believed medicine had a primary role in social reform, which he saw as "economic common sense." Welch's passion for scientific investigation persuaded him that prosperous communities had healthy residents who had good food, adequate shelter, and wages that permitted them to maintain these conditions. Lloyd C. Taylor Jr. described Welch as a proponent of "a radical program of social reform."

> He insisted that any successful attack on poverty must begin with the advancement of medical knowledge under the auspices of the federal government. The creation of a national government agency would provide the best means to coordinate the various municipal and state

bureaus. Since poverty represented an acute national issue, the federal government had a constitutional obligation to participate in the work.

Welch's interests were wide-ranging. He endorsed paved streets, construction of sewage systems, water purification projects, food inspection, and preventive medicine. More than half a century past his retirement, these ideas still ring with challenge for a society often willing to accept poverty and illness in the name of individualism and competition. Ever the researcher, Welch demonstrated to his own satisfaction that social reform and preventive medicine produced a better life for all people.[2]

Welch set a tone at Hopkins and recruited a faculty committed to his vision for medicine. They in turn trained some of the best and most conscientious physicians of the late nineteenth and early twentieth centuries. Although few of these reforming doctors came west to live, several became interested in the special maladies of working men and women. For example, William Osler, head of the Department of Medicine, became a leading tuberculosis researcher who advocated early diagnosis as the first step toward an eventual cure for the disease. Recognizing the costs of treating tubercular patients at sanitariums, he developed a scheme for home treatment, and his student Adelaide Dutcher documented the unsanitary habit of spitting, which transmitted the disease in public places and workplaces.[3] Working among poor sweatshop workers in Baltimore, Osler and Dutcher laid important foundations for what would become social and industrial medicine.

Another important ingredient in the emergence of scientific medicine with a social conscience was Abraham Flexner's muckraking study entitled *Medical Education in the United States and Canada* (1910), commonly referred to simply as the Flexner report. In his study of medical education Flexner described the status of medical education and especially criticized the proprietary schools whose purpose was to "make money." Although the report singled out the accomplishments of Johns Hopkins, Harvard, and Cornell, it presented a dismal portrait of other schools whose deans knew more about promotion than medicine. Influenced in emphasis by John Dewey and his project method, the Flexner report praised the scientific and ward-based education that marked the Johns Hopkins approach.[4]

No one more clearly demonstrated the influence of her Johns Hopkins training than America's preeminent industrial and social physician Dr. Alice Hamilton. Raised by nonconformist parents in rural Indiana, Dr. Hamilton spent two years at Miss Porter's School in Farmington, Connecticut, then attended the University of Michigan, where she encountered Richard Ely, the economist. From Michigan she went first to the New England Hospital for Women and then to Johns Hopkins Medical School, where she worked closely with Welch and Osler. She next went to Chicago's Hull House, which proved the perfect culmination to her preparation for industrial medicine. When she took up the study of America's most serious industrial disease, lead poisoning, her distinctive course intersected with the history of the U.S. mining industry and, ultimately, mining in the West.

As she became familiar with the status of industrial medicine in the United States, she learned that public sentiment associated it with socialism, and its practitioners were primarily substandard physicians employed by large corporations to protect themselves from industrial liability litigation. Beginning first with Illinois statistics, Dr. Hamilton became convinced that lead poisoning was a serious problem there. Her study singled out lead as a serious health hazard, in part because workers and managers presumed it was not a serious problem. The 1911 report documented that any contact whatsoever with lead fumes or dust contributed to the onset of the disease.

Smelters were obvious places of contact for workers, but so were print shops, white lead factories, paint factories and stores, battery factories, pottery and chamber pot factories, and commercial art studios. The bases for lead poisoning varied from smelter workers whose clothes and hair might be covered with lead dust to artists who carelessly sucked on their paintbrushes. Dr. Hamilton's studies of lead poisoning became the prototype for subsequent industrial health studies. When the Great War broke out in 1914, Hamilton discovered that wartime production gave sanitation new focus and added importance to her interest in industrial diseases.

In the aftermath of the infamous Arizona deportations in 1917, President Woodrow Wilson's mediation commission asked that Dr. Hamilton investigate conditions in the Arizona mining camps, which she did in early 1919. Among a host of grievances she discovered inequities between Mexican and U.S. miners, inadequate housing with neither fresh water nor sewage, and most important the widespread presence of miners' consumption. The disease was linked to the use of power drills and excessive dust underground; while some mines used wet drilling, this created its own hazards as men became soaked and thus more susceptible to colds and rheumatism. Other workers in the tank houses suffered from continuous exposure to poisonous gases, and their food absorbed the chemicals used to process the ores. Her findings in Arizona confirmed the link between mechanical drills and miners' consumption, demonstrated the prevalence of tuberculosis among the Mexican workers, and questioned the training and competence of the company doctors. She found the situation to be one in which labor and management were unable to reconcile their disagreements, which offered little promise for the individual miners.[5]

Dr. Hamilton's career in public health and industrial medicine brought eastern medical reformers into direct contact with western mining practices. Although she managed to shift national attention to the medical issues that plagued working miners, the miners themselves had spent considerable time and effort trying to remedy their concerns on their own. This record of self-help has been ably documented by Alan Derickson in his *Workers Health, Workers Democracy: The Western Miners' Struggle, 1891–1925*. Through the Western Federation of Miners (WFM) and their own health contracting, the miners employed strategies of self-help, collaboration with sympathetic or tolerant mining companies, and occasionally the creation of a parallel medical system miners could afford and depend on. According to Derickson twenty-five local WFM-affiliated unions created their own hospitals between 1897 and 1918.[6]

The WFM-sponsored hospitals were found in Telluride and Silverton, Colorado; Silver City, Idaho; Aldridge, Neihart, Gilt Edge, Kendall, and Zortman, Montana; Tonopah, Goldfield, Rhyolite, Manhattan, Beatty, Blair, Vernon, Round Mountain, and Rawhide, Nevada; Greenwater, California; Park City, Utah; and six in British Columbia. The miners created their own facilities because their alternative was usually to use locally retained physicians who entered into agreements with the dominant mining companies. Such arrangements were, as Hamilton noted, ordinarily designed to protect the mining company rather than to provide high-quality service to the individual miners who became patients. When and where the unions sponsored their own hospitals, they claimed the right to expend as they saw fit the medical fees, which companies charged against workers' wages. The medical men companies provided were often characterized as either novices willing to "work for a small salary and experience" or medical incompetents and social misfits. In any event, they were paid by the companies, which extracted their "retainers" from the wages of employees. As WFM locals created effective hospitals, new locals attempted to expand the practice to other communities. This pattern is most clearly illustrated in twentieth-century Nevada where unions created hospitals almost as soon as they were chartered. Derickson described these hospitals as "essentially residential in design."

> A common plan consisted of one or two general wards of four to eight beds each, along with a few private rooms for paying patients. Separate wards for infectious disease and maternity cases were exceptional. . . .
> The miners' institutions thus appear to have been western counterparts of the cottage hospitals of England and New England.[7]

Under Derickson's painstaking research into hospitals and political action, the WFM and its affiliates emerge as less radical and more practical than often characterized. They hired their own physicians, constructed hospitals, and engaged in extensive political pressure to ameliorate the working conditions and industrial diseases they recognized before experts such as Dr. Alice Hamilton. This recognition of the inherent dangers in their chosen vocation led miners to endorse workingmen's compensation legislation. Although workmen's comp gained broad support in the early twentieth century, occupational diseases such as silicosis were specifically excluded until near mid-century. Paradoxically, compensation for industrial diseases waited until mining as a vocation for Americans had entered a period of unalterable decline.[8]

In the early twentieth century both miners and companies became interested in applying new first-aid strategies to immediate care for injured miners. Although Derickson treats this concern as part of "the new paternalism," it undoubtedly benefited both miners and corporations that sponsored such programs. Both Arizona's Phelps Dodge mining operations and the American Smelting and Refining Company established safety programs modeled on one first developed at U.S. Steel between 1906 and 1911. The creation of the Bureau of Mines in 1911 also contributed to the new safety programs because the bureau was specifically denied enforcement authority. Arthur W. Page composed a fourteen-page article entitled " 'Safety First' Underground" for The World's Work in which he described the activities of the newly formed Bureau of Mines safety program. Page reported on the remarkable progress of the traveling mine safety cars and other educational programs in improving both mining practices and responses to actual emergencies.[9]

New concern for first aid built upon both growing public awareness of its utility and the obvious confidence its practitioners developed in time of crisis. In 1908 Arthur B. Reeve posed the question many critics were asking of U.S. industry, especially its mining industries: "Why not a 'Red Cross' for the Army of Industry?" According to Reeve, local medical practitioners gave rudimentary first-aid training to miners, who then employed the lessons in caring for their injured brethren. Rather like a group of scouts, Reeve described the meeting of first-aid teams who worked under the supervision of physicians and learned how to dress wounds and prepare the injured for removal to the doctor's office or a hospital. Given the unsanitary, ill-organized status of most underground stopes in early western mining, such instruction might have saved thousands of injured miners. Remembering briefly the Civil War surgeon's admonition to saw quickly, such training in prompt responses and proper care of injured men augured well for their recovery. One need only consider the alternatives—leaving the injured alone without treatment while seeking assistance or actually worsening the situation by attempting uniformed care and removal to get the injured to the doctor.[10]

Unquestionably, corporate management also benefited from safety programs, which addressed a series of identifiable problems that, if solved, often saved both time and money. One safety consultant explained precisely how he intended to use self-interest to transform a Phelps Dodge safety program during the 1920s.

> It is a basic principle of psychology that people are only mildly interested in what other people do for them, or at them; but they are intensely interested in the things that they do for themselves. . . . The secret of safety work is one of leading people to think, to act, and to talk safety, and not driving them to do so. Your problem of educating your people in safe thinking is indeed one of the hardest jobs imaginable. You are really trying to re-educate them, trying to help them to form entirely new habits, trying to get them to eradicate the chance taking habit and in its place to get them to cultivate the habit of being careful.[11]

For consultant H. H. Matthieson the safety program was an entirely new way of conceptualizing one's work and interaction with others. Although such instruction had traditionally been passed along to new employees by the skilled men who trained them or by supervisory personnel who introduced them to their work, miners learned work habits by observation and experience—precisely the areas safety programs wanted to alter. If workers did not practice and observe unsafe work habits, they would be less likely to employ them.

As early as 1906 the editor of *Mining Reporter* had made the same point in an essay entitled "Familiarity Breeds Contempt." He argued:

> There is a tendency to classify such errors as we have referred to according to the extent of their influence as measured by the number of people affected or the magnitude of the interest involved. For example, the loss of a single life caused by careless handling of explosives is by common consent considered of less consequence than the derangement of a metallurgical process due to a faulty calculation or analysis. In the former case, the consequences are meted out to the offending person only, while in the latter, interests other than those of the individual are made to pay the penalty of his carelessness.[12]

Both miners and management came to recognize that collective carelessness could produce disasters.

In one of the most poignant segments of his autobiography *Deep Enough*, Frank Crampton describes his work in 1908 in a Utah mine where the company entirely ignored safe practices. First, carelessness in the location and handling of powder occasioned a major explosion that killed a powder monkey, nippers, and the miners who were drawing powder. This event was serious, but the blast was so severe that it damaged the ground where the miners were working. Four days after the powder house explosion, the mine suffered a cave-in. Suddenly, Crampton and nineteen companions found themselves trapped underground. His description of his ten-day entombment is the classic account of this experience by an American. Among other difficulties, one of the men went insane; all starved, became chilled and then hypothermal, and spent days underground without light and alone with their thoughts. Crampton remembered vividly the moment when rescuers reached the entombed men.

> There was no chance of my putting anything over my eyes. I was so weak I couldn't move. . . . Then, as the stiffs who had worked to get to us came closer, we knew it was not a dream. And then I heard the sobs, deep-breathing sobs, trying to be held back, but breaking out nonetheless, for the strength to hold them back was gone. There I was sobbing, too, and tears running down and smarting under my tender-skinned face.[13]

Crampton spent nearly a month in a hospital recovering from the effects of injured legs and prolonged exposure that plagued him while waiting underground for his rescuers, and then he spent another three weeks under his doctor's care—almost two months lost to carelessness![14]

Although Crampton denounced the carelessness and callousness his former employers exhibited, he was fortunate that his accident occurred in 1909 rather than twenty or thirty years earlier. In an earlier time it would have been more difficult to assemble a voluntary rescue crew, who willingly worked night and day to rescue the nineteen survivors. Furthermore, there would not likely have been a hospital to convalesce in, and had there been, his convalescence might have become his death wake. Crampton lived and worked in a transitional era. Important research and soon thorough study of conditions underground or in the nearby mills and smelters would further improve miners' conditions, but there was evidence of some unqualified improvement as well as the degeneration of conditions caused by dry drilling.

Health care for injured miners had improved because real breakthroughs had occurred in medical science. Furthermore, medical training was being reexamined, and a small coterie of social physicians was advocating attention to the entire environment in which patients worked and lived. Improvements by the early 1900s would not compare with the changes that occurred in the next thirty years, but systematic attention to safety and first aid provided a dramatically different situation than the one encountered by the early Comstock miners who waited and festered for the physician, who would have to be brought underground if the man were to have the benefit of his generation's best medical care.

One major mine was a pioneer in industrial medicine—the Homestake in Lead, South Dakota, the country's leading gold producer. Back in

1877–1878 George Hearst, one of the mine's owners, had made a contract with a doctor, then established a hospital in the new camp for his workers, who paid a monthly fee. The Homestake expanded the program to cover families. Over the years a new building had been built, then improved and modernized. Hearst wanted to help make Lead a more attractive community for his workers and their wives and children.

Following George's death in 1891, his widow, Phoebe, expanded the program. By 1910 workers and their families received general medical, surgical, and obstetrical services free of charge. The company established an aid fund that paid benefits for both sickness and accidents, followed in 1917 by a pension system for longtime employees, those suffering from a physical disability, and widows of workers killed in accidents. These benefits were only part of a larger paternalistic program the Homestake established that made Lead one of the most attractive mining communities. Long before state and local governments provided such support, the Homestake showed the way.

As the Bureau of Mines (BOM) began to examine the conditions of miners after its creation in 1911, its officials gathered information and studied common problems. In 1917 G. H. Halberstadt described the BOM's understanding of its responsibilities, which he limited to training miners in safety and to affecting where possible the health and safety of miners in their communities. He then proceeded to explain the importance of first-aid training: "In rendering first-aid all that is necessary is to use common sense and to follow instructions. A first-aid man should not attempt work that should be done by a doctor or surgeon, but should simply make the patient comfortable."[15] Although this might have been characteristic of miners in all generations, earlier miners rarely even knew what practices to follow.

The influence of social and industrial medicine increased throughout the first two decades of the twentieth century. When combined with management concern with improved productivity, which identified time-lost accidents as serious problems, and the miners' determination to take matters such as their health and safety into their own hands if necessary, the future definitely held more promise than the past. Serious problems remained, none more important than the respiratory ailments, especially silicosis, that plagued underground miners. In some instances safety measures came quickly in the new era. Perhaps nothing more dramatically altered the hazards from falling rock than the widespread adoption after the Great War of the campaign helmet, now miner's hard hat. Generations of miners had sustained unnecessary head injuries because they refused to wear protective head gear. Suddenly, the widespread availability of surplus helmets persuaded companies and miners to adopt them as peacetime protection against rocks and dirt. The change occurred because miners, managers, and physicians collectively decided the helmets would make work safer. That trend became the characteristic feature of twentieth-century mining; collective safety became popular and profitable.

Notes

1. Lloyd C. Taylor Jr., *The Medical Profession and Social Reform, 1885–1945* (New York: St. Martin's, 1974), 2, as quoted in William H. Welch, "The Twenty-Fifth Anniversary of the Johns Hopkins Hospital," in W. C. Burket, ed., *Papers and Addresses of William Henry Welch*, 3 vols. (Baltimore: Johns Hopkins University Press, 1920), vol. 3, 25.

2. Taylor, *Medical Profession and Social Reform*, 3–4.

3. Taylor, *Medical Profession and Social Reform*, 30–32.

4. Abraham Flexner, *Medical Education in the United States and Canada: A Report to the Carnegie Foundation for the Advancement of Teaching*, Bulletin no. 4, Carnegie Foundation (Washington, D.C.: Science and Health Publications, 1960 [1910]); Taylor, *Medical Profession and Social Reform*, 45–46; Eugene Perry Link, *The Social Ideas of American Physicians 1776–1976: Studies in the Humanitarian Tradition in Medicine* (Selinsgrove, Penn.: Susquehanna University Press, 1992), 82; John Field, "Medical Education in the United States: Late Nineteenth and Early Twentieth Centuries," in C. D. O'Malley, ed., *The History of Medical Education; UCLA Forum in Medical Sciences*, no. 12 (Los Angeles: University of California Press, 1970), 506–510; and Martin Kaufman, *American Medical Education: The Formative Years, 1765–1910* (Westport, Conn.: Greenwood, 1976), 164–182.

5. Taylor, *Medical Profession and Social Reform*, 89–94.

6. Alan Derickson, *Workers' Health, Workers' Democracy: The Western Miners' Struggle, 1891–1925* (Ithaca: Cornell University Press, 1988), 57–101.

7. Derickson, *Workers' Health*, 101–121; quote 120.

8. Derickson, *Workers' Health*, 155–188.

9. Derickson, *Workers' Health*, 191–195; Arthur W. Page, "'Safety First' Underground," *The World's Work* 23 (March 1912), 549–556.

10. Arthur B. Reeve, "Why Not a 'Red Cross' for the Army of Industry?" *American Review of Reviews* 37 (February 1908), 201–203. See also Augustin H. Goelet, M.D., "How to Deal With Apparent Death From Electric Shock," *Scientific American* (November 3, 1894), 281–282; J. C. Royle, "Mine Rescue Cars in Action," *Colliers* 46 (January 21, 1911), 20.

11. H. H. Matthieson, Consulting Engineer, "Report on the Copper Queen Branch of Phelps Dodge Corporation," May 1928, 1–2 in Safety File, Box 58, Frank A. Ayer Collection, American Heritage Center, Laramie, Wyoming.

12. "Familiarity Breeds Contempt," *Mining Reporter* 53, 2 (November 11, 1906), 24.

13. Frank Crampton, *Deep Enough: A Working Stiff in the Western Mine Camps* (Denver: Sage, 1956), 105–116, quote 116.

14. Crampton, *Deep Enough*, 118–121.

15. G. H. Halberstadt et al., *Advanced First-Aid Instructions for Miners: A Report on Standardization* (Washington, D.C.: Government Printing Office, 1917), 3–5, quote 5.

Bibliographic Essay

OR THOSE INTERESTED IN SPECIFIC REFERENCES, we refer you to the foot-
notes. This essay provides a general overview of sources in two sec-
tions—urban and industrial.

Urban

A bonanza of general and specific American medical histories has appeared
since around 1975. Although most touch only briefly on the West and little,
if at all, on mining, the following provide excellent overviews: James H.
Cassedy, *Medicine in America* (Baltimore: Johns Hopkins University Press,
1991); John Duffy, *The Healers: A History of American Medicine* (Urbana:
University of Illinois Press, 1976); John S. Haller Jr., *American Medicine in
Transition 1840–1910* (Urbana: University of Illinois Press, 1981); Charles
E. Rosenberg, *The Care of Strangers* (New York, Basic, 1987); and Paul Starr,
The Social Transformation of American Medicine (New York: Basic, 1982).

More specialized studies touch upon a variety of topics. A list of those
that provide fascinating insights includes James G. Burrow, *AMA: Voice
of American Medicine* (Baltimore: Johns Hopkins University Press, 1963);
Martin Kaufman, *American Medical Education* (Westport, Conn.: Greenwood, 1976); David and Elizabeth Armstrong, *The Great American Medicine
Show* (New York; Prentice-Hall, 1991); Kenneth Allen De Ville, *Medical
Malpractice in Nineteenth-Century America* (New York: New York University
Press, 1990); Kenneth M. Ludmerer, *Learning to Heal: The Development of
American Medical Education* (Baltimore: Johns Hopkins University Press,
1985); and William G. Rothstein, *American Medical Schools and the Practice
of Medicine* (New York: Oxford University Press, 1987).

A general medical history of the West is still awaited. James Breeden,
ed., *Medicine in the West* (Manhattan: Sunflower University Press, 1982),
a special issue of *Journal of the West*, provides a fine start. The researcher
should go to the broader medical histories or specific studies to find needed
background. For example, see Thomas Hall, *Medicine on the Santa Fe Trail*

(Dayton: Morningside, 1971); Robert Karolevitz, *Doctors of the Old West* (Seattle: Superior, 1967); Clarence Meyer, *American Folk Medicine* (New York: Thomas Y. Crowell, 1973); Elizabeth Van Steenwyk, *Frontier Fever* (New York: Walker, 1995); and Alfred W. Crosby Jr., *Epidemic and Peace, 1918* (Westport, Conn.: Greenwood, 1976).

Several state medical histories have been published that contain varied amounts of information on mining; for example, Henry Harris, *California's Medical Story* (San Francisco: Grabborn, 1932); Paul Phillips, *Medicine in the Making of Montana* (Missoula: Montana State University Press, 1962); Frances Quebbeman, *Medicine in Territorial Arizona* (Phoenix: Arizona Historical Foundation, 1966); Jake Spidle Jr., *Doctors of Medicine in New Mexico* (Albuquerque: University of New Mexico Press, 1986); and Robert H. Shikes, *Rocky Mountain Medicine: Doctors, Drugs, and Diseases in Early Colorado* (Boulder: Johnson, 1986).

Most histories of mining towns and camps mention medical topics; this is true of both nineteenth- and twentieth-century publications. The recent accounts are more likely to utilize a thorough scholarly approach to the subject. Some of the early state histories, such as the Bancroft volumes and others, had accounts of epidemics and doctors and a variety of information.

Although fewer historical medical articles on the West have been written than might be hoped, a start has been made. Again, this will take time and patience looking through state historical journals and other publications and more specialized medical works. A few dissertations also focus on medicine; see particularly Leanne L. Sander, "The Men All Died of Miners' Disease: Women and Families in the Industrial Mining Environment of Upper Clear Creek Colorado, 1870–1900," unpublished Ph.D. dissertation, University of Colorado, 1990.

Primary sources remain the best way to gain a feel for the time and place. A few doctors have left reminiscences: E. W. Too, ed., *A Doctor on the California Trail* (Denver: Old West, 1971); Charles Gardiner, *Doctor at Timberline* (Caldwell: Caxton, 1938); and Kenneth Johnson, ed., *The Gold Rush Letters of J.D.B. Stillman* (Palo Alto: Lewis Osborne, 1967) are fine places to start. In *The Shirley Letters* (numerous editions), Louise Clapp blends a wonderful account of her doctor-husband and a woman's view of life in the camp.

There are sundry firsthand accounts by people who lived and worked in the mining towns. Almost all of these make some reference to medicine or illness, and although it may take effort to find the nuggets, they are there. The researcher can learn about both male and female attitudes and concerns and look at large towns and small, isolated camps. Add to this the unpublished journals, letters, and reminiscences that can be found in archives, historical societies, and libraries throughout the West. Photographs also contribute special flavor, although few deal with mining camp medical subjects.

The same general observation is true for the mining camp newspapers, a bonanza of information about all aspects of medicine. It takes sharp reading, but the exertion is worth it; the researcher must keep in mind, however, that occasionally diseases and epidemics are downplayed for fear of hurting a community's image.

State medical publications and a variety of government (local, state, and federal) publications provide a wide range of information and statistics. States also published pamphlets praising their virtues, including medical, although some claims must be taken with a grain of salt. The material is out there waiting to be prospected in this relatively untapped field of western history.

Index